HEALTH

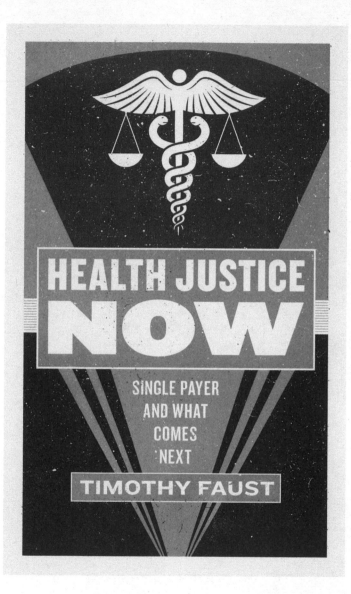

HEALTH JUSTICE NOW

SINGLE PAYER AND WHAT COMES NEXT

TIMOTHY FAUST

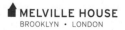

MELVILLE HOUSE
BROOKLYN · LONDON

HEALTH JUSTICE NOW

Copyright © 2019 by Timothy Faust
First Melville House Printing: August 2019

Melville House Publishing   Suite 2000
                46 John Street   and   16/18 Woodford Rd.
        Brooklyn, NY 11201   London E7 0HA

mhpbooks.com
@melvillehouse

ISBN: 978-1-61219-716-6
ISBN: 978-1-61219-717-3 (eBook)

Printed in the United States of America

10 9 8 7 6 5 4 3 2 1

A catalog record for this book is available from the Library of Congress

To Kelly Jo,

who pulls me from the swamp

and breathes life into me

Also to Ronnie James Dio

CONTENTS

Part IV: What We Do

HEALTH JUSTICE NOW

A secret scream rings through America. It rings down the sterile fluorescent hallways of our hospitals. It rings over our rural towns and our Native reservations. It rings through our prisons, the bellies of our great American cities. It rings in our farms and our fields, our streets and our sewers, our bodies and our blood, and we are cursed to never hear it clearly until, at last, we realize it has been our own mouth screaming, and we are lost. A child born today inherits in that secret a new American squalor, the skeletal remains of the American cities, the bleached bones of the American suburbs. This secret is a birthright of continual exploitation, pumped for labor and drained of cash and then punished for the resulting suffering— punished for being hungry, punished for being sick, punished for being pregnant, punished for being poor, punished for being black or brown, for being queer, for being unlucky, for *being*.

At the base of that suffering is lodged a little truth, like a knot in the stomach: in America, sickness makes you poor; and poorness makes you sick.

This is a book about that relationship, and why it happens, and why it's unnecessary and what we can do to fix it. The cosmic whirling of God's great slot machine has not determined that some people are fated to suffer while others flourish. We have the resources to take care of everyone, and yet we refuse to do so. Your medical debt and medical bills are unnecessary, but we have chosen to make them necessary. These are structural problems with structural causes, and many of them share roots in how we pay for healthcare.

This is a book about healthcare and health finance. They are different. Healthcare is anything that helps you stay safe and healthy. It is a kind of freedom from, and within, your own body. Health finance is the method by which we, as a country, pay for that freedom, and by which we decide who gets to have it, and who doesn't. Healthcare is more than what happens to you in the hospital. Healthcare is whether your home makes you sick or your food makes you sick or your environment makes you sick or whether you have enough money to afford the things that keep you healthy. In America, the structure of corporate health finance has convinced us that some people deserve healthcare, and some people don't.

This is a book about that corporate health finance—about private insurance and private insurers. For a half century, they've convinced us that they are the only things that keep us—that could *ever* keep us—from the utter financial ruination of illness. They've sold us different inadequate insurance plans and persuaded us that this is a form of great liberty, while chipping away at our freedoms for profit, and holding our bodies and our children's bodies hostage.

This is a book about single-payer healthcare, a health finance model in which we pool our abundant collective resources to provide healthcare to all people. It is a common model across the world. As we will discuss in this book, we have the potential not just to enact a single-payer program in America but to build the greatest healthcare program among any so-called developed country.

Here is my profession of faith:

I believe beyond any doubt that single-payer is demonstrably sound and eminently feasible. I believe a properly ambitious and well-structured single-payer program will do more than any other American social program of this generation to soothe the burns, to resuscitate the spirit, to nourish the moral will of the American people. I believe it will loosen the loathsome manacles of American health finance: an exploitative institution that profits by plundering from us our own bodily autonomy and that anchors a larger exploitation, that holds those whom we love as captive leverage to guarantee our servitude to abusive employers or domestic partners—to those who seek to dominate us both in the office and in the hospital.

I believe this nation owes its people, whose labor has created its rich banquet, the safety and agency of healthcare. I believe this healthcare is greater in scope than that which happens upon an operating table. I believe that housing, food, income, and more—the components of basic human dignity—are healthcare, and I believe our work is that of striving toward justice for all people; and I therefore believe—I have to believe—that single-payer healthcare is our moral imperative. Single payer is our tool. Single payer is our weapon. Single payer is our first step. But single payer, on its own, is not the goal.

This is a book about health justice.

★   ★   ★

Healthcare is personal. So I want to start this book personally by introducing two friends of mine, Steve Way and Kyle Kolich. They're two guys about my age (I'm 30) who live in north New Jersey. They're sweet, gentle people and probably the most charismatic pair of friends I've met in my entire life. They make me laugh until my face hurts, and we like watching pro wrestling together. They're also being utterly broken by our American health system, and it's keeping them from living their lives.

Steve has muscular dystrophy. The muscles and tissues that hold his body together are eating themselves. He's doing pretty good, all things considered. He beat his original life expectancy of 18 and now probably has a long life ahead of him.

Steve needs a wheelchair to move and a ventilator to help him breathe. He also needs help getting dressed, going to the bathroom, eating, and other everyday functions. His family takes care of him, but Steve doesn't want to be dependent on his parents for his whole life. He wants to move in with his girlfriend. But Steve can't afford to hire a private personal medical assistant 24/7. I mean, who could?

In many parts of the United States, if you can't receive care at home, you have to live in a nursing home (or an SNF, a skilled nursing facility). Nursing homes are private institutions for people who can't live on their own, like people with disabilities and senior citizens with advanced medical needs. But many people do not want to live in a nursing home. Caregivers are massively overworked and deeply underpaid, and the result is often shallow, loveless care, with high rates of medical negligence. Nursing homes have been caught bribing judges to reduce their medical malpractice lawsuit damages, sending their own corporate officials to run for office (who then make it harder to file a malpractice case), or hiring their own lawmakers directly as employees.[1] These are not good prospects for someone who needs medical care, nor for someone who wants to be permitted to live freely instead of being imprisoned in a warehouse. "Nursing homes are where [people like me] go to die," Steve says.

Because Steve wants to avoid all of this, he needs Medicaid. Medicaid is an insurance program, funded jointly by federal and state governments, for people who don't make much money and people with disabilities. Medicaid pays for much of Steve's healthcare, and also a home-health budget, which he can use to pay home-health aides to come over a set number of hours a week and assist him around the house. Home-health aides help Steve move, cook, clean, refresh his meds, and stay healthy. They mean he can lead the life he wants to, like all of us do.

But not all state Medicaid programs pay for home health, and few of them pay for it in the same way. Paid or not, the work must be done. For most of his life, Steve's family, especially his mother, has pitched in to take care of his health needs. Being able to receive care at home makes Steve incredibly lucky.

Getting Medicaid to pitch in took a long time. A few years ago, after a lot of phone calls, paperwork, appointments, and waiting, New Jersey Medicaid approved Steve's request for home-health funding. Some people hire external home-health aides using Medicaid, but Steve was able to use this money to hire his mother so she could be compensated for some of her help. This took some of the sting out of her not being able to work as many hours as she might otherwise like to outside the house. Then came Kyle.

Kyle and Steve's friendship started before they were born: Kyle's mom and Steve's dad have been friends since middle school. Kyle and Steve started hanging out and writing sketch comedy together sometime between high school and college.

Kyle decided to go to acting school in New York, then met his wife and settled in Astoria, Queens. A year later, his back gave out while he was putting groceries into the bottom shelf of his refrigerator. The injury kept him from his bartending jobs for a week, which (as most working people know) is a devastating amount of money to lose out on. It happened again—another back injury, another wageless week. Then things got complicated.

Kyle contracted parvovirus in his knee, which meant he racked up a substantial amount of medical debt and missed more work. While he was recovering, his wife, Rivera, a Canadian citizen who had just received her working papers after months of being prohibited from working in the United States, developed a kidney infection and had to be rushed to the emergency room. More medical debt—major medical debt. A mountain of debt that just about exhausted everything Kyle and Rivera had, and then some: a total bulldozing that took only six months from start to finish.

So Kyle and Rivera moved in with Kyle's parents back in Jersey to save up money and pay off their debt. Since he lived just down the road, Kyle spent more time at Steve's. This was good. They got to hang out, and Kyle would help Steve, meaning Steve's mom got a break. One day, Steve turned to Kyle and said, "Man, you already help me take a shit. You might as well get paid for it." Steve reallocated his home-health budget to hire Kyle, who now was paid to take care of his friend.

That's a charming plot point. But it keeps getting worse. Both Steve and Kyle are getting squeezed in different ways by American health finance.

Steve has to fight for every hour of home health he gets. Originally, Medicaid approved him for 35 hours of paid home health. Steve needs much more than 40 hours of home health. He needs more than 50 hours of weekly home health. He's a person, not a nine-to-five construction job.* After years of negotiating, that budget slowly rose—to 36, to 37, to 38. Eventually it was raised to 40, but nobody told Steve about it, and once he found out from an unrelated encounter with the Medicaid office, the payments weren't retroactive.

To qualify for this home-health budget, a nurse comes to Steve's house every four months. Her job is to confirm that Steve is "still" disabled. Both she and Steve understand that this is a useless interaction: Steve weighs maybe 45 pounds sopping wet—he's not getting out of that wheelchair. But Medicaid wants to make sure he's not trying to scam them, so he has to go through this process over and over and over again. Miss an appointment, mess up, or get the paperwork wrong, and Kyle doesn't get paid.

Kyle needs this money to pay off his medical bills and, maybe one day, move back to Queens. He, too, would prefer not to live with his parents for the rest of his life (and his wife, I

---

* Jersey's Medicaid program had just decided that, for Steve, the time beyond 40 hours isn't worth compensating.

presume, would certainly enjoy a break from the in-laws). But Kyle is only paid 11 bucks an hour. He's not even getting Steve's full 40 hours a week, since Steve allocates part of his home-health budget to his mother and girlfriend, so they get essential compensation for the time they spend with him while Kyle wasn't around.* Kyle ultimately had to take a second job in retail just so he could get health insurance—there's a shortage of home-health providers in America, driven in part by how low the wages are, and people can't even take care of their friends or loved ones without being punished for it.

And speaking of wages: Steve is a substitute teacher. I've never seen him teach, but I've seen him speak, and he's good at it. If Steve wants to stay out of a nursing home, however, he is not allowed to work as many shifts as he'd like. The state of New Jersey has decided that home health is only subsidized for people . . . who make less than $2,000 a year! If Steve works more than a few shifts in a month, he becomes ineligible.

Here's what this means: Steve has to hope he can keep jumping through incredible bureaucratic hoops if he wants to stay alive. People who want to help Steve are forced to drop out of the job market and receive appallingly low wages just so the person they love doesn't die. Steve's family has been punished by Medicaid, because two of its members, both Steve and his mom, can't work, even though they both can and would like to.† And Kyle isn't paid enough to pay off his own medical debt. Kyle has to choose between taking care of his friend and having his own health insurance. Nobody is happy. My friends are being hosed. All the reasons for it are arbitrary and degrading.

This anecdote isn't meant to show how particularly unlucky Steve and Kyle are. They're not. They're regular unlucky. This is the American healthcare system working as normal: this is

---

* Plus the dozens and dozens of unpaid, uncompensated hours Steve's girl-friend, mother, and Kyle spend with him.

† Though, of course, one's worthiness of healthcare, shelter, food, or safety shouldn't be dependent on one's compatibility with the workforce.

just what happens if you're sick, or injured, or have a disability, or are poor, or are black or brown. The disability community uses the phrase "temporarily able-bodied" to describe people presently without disabilities. It's a good term. No matter how healthy you are now, eventually something—a car you're driving, a car you're not, a slippery surface, a genetic mutation—won't break your way. When that happens, you usually end up in debt, in a hospital, or trapped at home.

The problem isn't that Steve and Kyle are *unlucky*. The problem is that to avoid their fates, you have to be extremely *lucky*.

★   ★   ★

Healthcare is personal, *micropersonal* even, because it happens both to us and within us. We've all felt hassled or harassed by contemporary American healthcare and health finance. I happen to know a little more than most people. In 2014, I wrote code to help find people to enroll in the Affordable Care Act (ACA) in Florida, Georgia, and Texas—all "Medicaid gap" states, in which folks fell in the gulf between ACA and Medicaid eligibility—and knocked on doors to talk to people in Orlando. There, I spent most of my time meeting people who just didn't *qualify* for the ACA because their states didn't expand Medicaid. They were too poor, or they were the wrong kind of poor. This broke my brain a little—how could these elected officials refuse to expand Medicaid and thus actively harm a lot of their constituents? Couldn't the ACA *still* work somehow? It was so big and complicated! What was insurance, anyway? How can we make it work for everybody?

To learn more, I took a job in the insurance industry, building little tools for nurses to look at a map and learn who had diabetes and who didn't, thinking the ACA could work if it *just* had the resources it needed.

I was wrong, humiliatingly wrong, absolutely wrong without fail, and this book is my attempt at penance.

I wanted to know more about these needs; I wanted to learn more about the brutal delta between the fantasy and the reality. I read papers, I read books, I did all the nerd shit, but that's not enough to really understand how healthcare needs manifest. Health disparity is local. There is a world of difference between health needs in Boston, Birmingham, Brooklyn, and Boise. So I took to the road.

Over the past two years, I've driven around the United States in my 2002 Honda CR-V* as a healthcare justice speaker. I've spoken in almost every continental state, in big cities and small ones. I've met people who are fighting to get their communities what they deserve, I've met people who are just curious about how insurance works, I've met people who are winning major legislative battles, I've met people who have had great harm inflicted upon them. It is always the same, every morning on the road: I wake up and drive six hours, get to a new town, give my speech, and answer as many questions as I can. Then somebody walks up to me and shares with me the worst thing that has ever happened to them. I have become a library of the miseries of strangers. It is an honor to be trusted with such personal stories.

Through it all, I have seen such suffering.

I have been welcomed into families thrust into inescapable debt because of complications from pregnancy. I have met the children whose birth caused that debt, the children who were born *into* that debt, who will carry it all their lives—whose birthright is a tiny pair of manacles, forged within hospital billing departments.

I have sat with widows and widowers, people who watched those whom they love writhe in agony in hospital beds; who, out of love, spent everything they had to try to ameliorate that agony; who failed and who were failed; and who now carry themselves in both heartbreak and poverty.

---

* 300,000 miles!

I have met people who were born into bodies that suffer; I have wept in front of them as they share with me the depth of the dehumanization forced upon them, whose daily existence is a constant blaring reminder that they are not wanted, who are forced to make an occupation out of begging over and over again for basic help.

I have visited wealthy hospital campuses for wealthy hospital patients, virtual islands in the middle of their cities. I have visited the neighborhoods around them—black and brown neighborhoods systematically drained of capital and labor in a dance reminiscent of colonialism, who, too poor to receive care at the hospital, in many cases, made poor *by* the hospital and its growth and economic power, suffer and die much, much sooner than the people in wealthier neighborhoods just a few miles away.

I've visited rural towns and rural counties, where there are few doctors and fewer hospitals, where people watch friends and places slip away, where cratering home prices mean nobody can afford to leave and the job famine means nobody can afford to return, where suicide rates are high and car accidents, so far away from an emergency room, often mean death.

And, over time, I have felt my own body betray me. I have looked in the mirror and seen my own coming crisis. I myself am a sick man, heir to my family's mental illness, and by it I am bedridden at least a quarter of the year. I have paced miles around my city block fearing the decay of my own temporary able-bodiedness and the wave of punishments—the punishments for the sin of being sick—in which I am eventually going to drown.

But it does not do justice to the people I've met to pornographize their suffering. It is insufficient to simply recite a litany of human pain. This book exists thanks to those who shared their suffering with me, in the long, long hope that we, together, can build the world in which nobody need suffer in the way they have.

But why does it happen? Why does American healthcare, which is a savior to so many, crush so many more under its heel? Why do bad things happen to good people—to whom bad things have already happened?

This is a book for people who have felt pushed around, knocked down, or fucked over by the American health finance system. This is a book that will attempt to explain why you can't afford to go to the doctor, why your doctor can't afford to see you, and who's making money off your misery. It is a book for those who see this suffering burned into the mirror, or into the faces of the people they love, and who are sick as hell of the whole thing. This is, I hope, a book for everyone who wants something better.

My aim over the course of this book is to explain why all this came to be and why it happens the way it does. I'll start with what we got: what co-pays are, for example; what insurance itself is; why healthcare costs increase so steeply; or why the few remaining rural hospitals and clinics close at such an alarming rate. Then, in part two, I'll talk about both *a)* what we want instead, which is comprehensive, robust single-payer insurance in America—which you might know as "Medicare for All"— and *b)* the inadequate options we're currently being offered.

But that's only a fragment of our story. In the third part of this book, I'll discuss how single-payer is only a smaller piece of our larger goal. I want readers of this book to understand that access to insurance only represents a small portion—approximately a fifth[2]—of the health inequalities in the United States. I want you to understand that most health disparity comes from things like inadequate or unsafe housing, inadequate or unsafe food, lack of income or lack of safety. And I want you to understand that these things don't just "happen"—people don't just "happen" to have nuclear waste buried in their backyards; poor people don't just "happen" to live in crumbling death traps. These things are caused by structural poverty and structural racism, by patriarchal, economic, and racial domination.

Against these monsters, insurance alone is not enough.

So if we hope for a world in which nobody is made to suffer, in which people like Steve, Kyle, you, and me, and everyone we know, can feel safe inside our own bodies—we must expand our vision of the fight. We must conceive of the fight for single-payer as one among many in pursuit of *health justice*. We must fight the battles to help people who are suffering now, and, with those victories, create the scaffolding of a single-payer movement aimed toward health justice. The history of the fight for health reform tells us that we can afford nothing else.

PART I:

WHAT WE GOT

PART I: WHAT WE GOT

What is "healthcare in America"? It's huge, and it's been made hard to understand, and depending upon where you were born and to whom, it either saves or ruins your life.

It's a machine so big, almost cosmic in scope, that you can't see all of it in one field of view. It's an infinitely cascading network of relationships between hundreds of millions of people—not just you and your doctor, but you and your family, you and your landlord, you and the person who sells you food, you and the police, you and the city planner who decided whether a bus runs near your house, and the thousands of relationships *they* have—your doctor and the dozens and dozens of pharmaceutical and equipment salespeople who visit your doctor's office, for example.

We learn about healthcare in fits and bursts. A lot of us learn from firsthand experience. The American ideal is a smooth process: you feel unwell, so you go to the doctor, who gives you some medicine—or who sends you to another doctor who better knows what to do. Eventually, after receiving care paid for by your insurance (plus a small fee put aside for you to pay), you feel better.

That's rarely how it works. Too many of us try to do the right thing—go to a doctor, be very careful, check all the boxes, and read all the fine print—and find ourselves with more medical costs than we could ever hope to afford. And then we're stung. The next time we feel something *wrong* inside of us, we're too afraid to ask anyone what to do about it. We panic, and in that panic we make choices that end up costing us even more dearly.

But how did it get this way? Hell, what *is* "this way"? Here is the state of the nation that American health finance has given us:

- America spends more than any other country on healthcare*—almost twice as much per capita as other wealthy countries[1]—while caring little about community health, caring little about population health, caring little about that which cannot be packaged and sold.
- 75 percent of our spending goes to chronic conditions that are preventable, yet nobody paying the bills really has tried to prevent them.[2]
- Our system of for-profit private insurers literally takes money from poor people and gives it to wealthy people. It is negatively redistributive. In 2014 it pushed millions of people into poverty or extreme poverty.[3]

What a rotten structure. It's certainly affected you personally, but health finance is wrapped up in so many other different things that it hides itself within other problems, like a Russian nesting doll of wretchedness. Maybe you recognize it if you have, or have had, one of these questions:[†]

- Why am I in so much medical debt?
- Why does it cost so much to go to the doctor?
- Why did my ER bill include $40 for bandages?
- Why can I only go to some doctors but not others?

---

*   I'm not necessarily upset about the amount of money America spends on healthcare. I'm upset at how *badly* it's being spent, and how many people don't benefit from it.

†   If you haven't (lucky you!), someone you love certainly has.

- Why are people with disabilities forced into nursing homes?
- Why do I still get billed by the hospital even when I'm insured?
- What the hell is an insurance premium, and why do they go up every year?
- Why does my boss tell me I can't get a raise because my healthcare costs have gone up?

There's one simple answer to all of these questions: *you're being exploited*. You're being taken advantage of. To put it bluntly, you're being fucked over.

The method of the exploitation, the precise rules and regulations by which you're being needled, and the artfulness of the cover-up vary from person to person and neighborhood to neighborhood. But ultimately, American healthcare means you're made sick, and then punished for being sick, all so someone else can turn a huge profit.

Maybe you already knew that but want to know the *why* and *how*. Over the next few pages, I'm going to attempt to describe American healthcare thoroughly enough to answer each of these questions. Let's explore the wet 'n' wild world of American health finance together.

★   ★   ★

The most fundamental fact of American healthcare is that nobody, except for mega-millionaires, can afford to pay for their healthcare costs out of pocket.*

---

* Mega-millionaires can not only afford to pay for their own medical costs, but there are entire hospitals with luxury wings specifically *for* these extravagantly wealthy people. While I believe in the essential dignity of being human, I am not very concerned about the healthcare of people making tens of millions of dollars a year. They'll be fine.

Medical costs don't affect us all evenly, and they don't all hit us at the same time. Half of all medical costs in the United States in a given year come from only 5 percent of patients.[4] And four fifths of medical costs come from one fifth of all American patients.[5] In a given year, some people have million-dollar hospital bills, some people have $300,000 medications, and some people get into major car accidents or need heart surgery, while most other people don't.

This only measures American *patients*—that is, people who were able to access or afford a doctor in the first place. There are without a doubt billions of dollars in medical costs that do not get spent because the would-be patients don't have insurance and don't go to the doctor because of it, or because they *do* have insurance but can't afford to use it. Being unable to afford healthcare prevents you from becoming a patient in the first place. This creeps into your psyche: we know, for example, that people with less money report fewer of their illnesses.[6]

These patient populations aren't usually the same people every single year. While a lot of people have significant medical costs every year—maybe they're older or have a disability or need expensive medication to stay alive—generally speaking, costs move around from person to person. Some years you might be off the hook and have few medical costs. Other years you might give birth to a baby or get hit by a car or have a heart attack—then it's your turn on the table. And when it is, you almost certainly won't be able to pay for it out of pocket. Having a child, for example, can be billed at anywhere between $32,000 and $50,000,[7] though it sometimes reaches into the *millions* of dollars—it's hard to get out of the natal intensive care unit (NICU) with less than a $500,000 bill—with no way to predict costs before you land in the delivery room. If you don't want to leave with a six-figure bill, you need **insurance**.*

---

*   You may still leave with a six-figure bill.

INSURANCE

For a long time, out-of-pocket spending, or paying a doctor directly from your own wallet, was the only way people in America paid for their healthcare—though the quality of that "healthcare" has changed dramatically over time. While some workers in Germany had a form of insurance beginning in the 1890s,* America took its sweet time getting there.

For as long as America has been around, there have been people who couldn't afford healthcare—or who couldn't afford anything at all. Throughout the 1800s and into the 1900s, poorhouses sprung up across the country. They were short- and long-term refuges for the poor, and they expected hard labor in return. Only if a person was physically unable to perform work were they permitted to be left alone.

Poorhouses were filthy, brutal bunkhouses that existed at the knife-edge between American charity and Puritan work ethics. Poverty must be made so utterly miserable, and relief must be made so meager, that work—any kind of work—is preferable by comparison. This ideology, of punishing the unproductive, has never really left America. We've just practiced hiding it.

Then there's medicine. In the early 1900s, rich families would pay doctors for private care in their homes,[8] poor people might go to a fledgling hospital and hope for charity palliative care, and millions of Americans lived somewhere in the middle. But medicine was wildly unregulated, medical standards were virtually nonexistent, and quality of care oscillated dramatically from doctor to doctor. As a result, healthcare costs were very low, and usually only borne by people who could

---

* The German insurance model of the 1890s was implemented, you may note, only because Otto von Bismarck was so afraid of socialists that he passed an insurance program for low-income workers to take the wind out of their sails and lessen their popular support.

afford them and who wanted to offset the costs of not being able to work because of illness. Healthcare was thus rationed out according to wealth and, usually, by race.

Millions of people still couldn't access any healthcare at all. Patients waited in long lines at public hospitals or public clinics, waiting for prescriptions they couldn't afford to fill. Often, hospitals would subject patients to grueling interviews to determine how expensive their care would be to provide. Too expensive, and the patients were denied entry.[9]

With the development and advancement of the hospital, and corresponding advances in quality of care, came the rapid growth of healthcare costs.* By the early 1930s, a family who sought medical care might find that hospital costs represented 40 percent of their total bill[10] (up from 15 percent a few years before).[11] But hospitals had a lot of capacity, hospital beds were going empty, and hospitals were interested in finding ways to fill them—by marketing themselves as the place where a person ought to have their children, for example. These schemes fell short in the face of the Depression, when suddenly *nobody* could afford healthcare, and hospital beds across the country stayed empty.

Some hospitals and some patients fared better. In the decade before the Depression, the Baylor University Hospital in Dallas, Texas, struck a deal with a local teachers' group: pay 50 cents a month in premiums, and Baylor would cover the cost

---

*   That hospitals are the primary locus of American health finance discussion is no accident. Much of the momentum that existed for national insurance after World War II was ceded by Harry S. Truman and other powerful Democrats in the face of opposition by industry and racist Southern Democrats. Instead, it was funneled into a bipartisan and industry-friendly movement to massively subsidize the creation of hospitals across the country—the Hill-Burton act of 1946. Hill-Burton built hundreds of new hospitals with public money but made no to attempt to exert any control over the business of those hospitals—a conscious choice encouraged by the anti-regulatory American Medical Association (AMA) and other anti–national insurance lobbies. Hill-Burton hospitals were thus permitted to use their public funding to offer segregated care or refuse care to the poor.

of any hospitalization. After the Depression hit and other hospitals couldn't attract paying patients, Baylor (and its teachers) were safe. The non-paying patients waited in the forever-long hospital lines, while doctors demanded the government subsidize the care they would otherwise be giving (and losing money on) for free. But this Baylor insurance model was successful for the patients who were included in it and kept the Baylor Hospital revenue running. Later, this insurance plan spun off into its own organization, called Blue Cross.

A decade later, during World War II, American factories were having a hard time attracting employees and distinguishing themselves as benevolent employers during a wage freeze. In 1943, the Internal Revenue Service ruled that health insurance was a fringe benefit and therefore tax-free. This meant employers could now offer competitive insurance plans to sidestep the wage freeze and lure in new workers. Families joined these plans rapidly, as Melissa Thomasson, a historian at Miami University of Ohio, has noted: the insured American population grew from 9 percent in 1940 to 63 percent in 1953, reaching 70 percent by the 1960s.[12]

Teachers, a hospital marketing scheme, WWII, and tax credits: from these components sprawl the massive, ramshackle American health insurance machine. It's a giant machine and it wasn't designed very well. In fact, it wasn't designed *at all*—there was no master plan behind the architecture. It was assembled piece by unknowable piece, bandage by unmeasurable bandage, without any sort of blueprint and thus it contains many moving parts performing strange and uncoordinated tasks. How you interact with it depends on a lot of things—whether you live in an urban or rural area, whether you're old or young, whether you're poor or wealthy, whether you're a member of the armed services, and what type of insurance you may or may not have. We'll go through each kind of insurance, one at a time.

UNINSURANCE

Some people—too many people—confront this machine without any insurance at all: 15.5 percent, or more than one in seven people, are uninsured.[13] This number is disproportionately higher among poor people—poverty and **uninsurance** go hand in hand.[14] Uninsured people are responsible for paying all the costs of going to the doctor or visiting a hospital—if they even make it to the hospital in the first place. Because the costs of receiving healthcare so greatly exceed what most people can ever hope to afford, even if those people aren't poor, hospitals typically decline to serve people who are uninsured (though they're legally required to stabilize, not treat, people in immediate mortal danger).* Otherwise, you're on your own: hope there's a free clinic nearby, or a sliding-scale community clinic.†

It's just awful to be uninsured. You're significantly less likely to have diseases like cancer diagnosed before they're severe, you're more likely to die from any given medical condition or disease, and you get less and worse care in the hospital even if you're admitted.[15] Choices like "medicine or rent?" or "healthy food or a doctor's visit?" are urgent and deeply infuriating in their obvious injustice—but what can you do about it? Just one accidental injury—like just one engine failure, or just one parking ticket—can knock over everything you've worked so hard to put together. If you ever fall sick, the deep and unknowable awfulness of medical costs—*How much is this going*

---

* Hospitals are also required to treat people who are in labor, though certain Catholic hospitals have really abused the boundaries of these requirements and will deny care to patients presenting with a stillbirth or miscarriage, afraid of providing an abortion, until the patient is in critical condition. See https://www.aclu.org/sites/default/files/field_document/growth-of-catholic-hospitals-2013.pdf.

† I would like to personally thank the Haight Ashbury Free Clinic in San Francisco for taking care of me in the years 2009–2010, when I had less than $100 to my name and also swine flu.

to cost? Can I put this on a credit card? Can I get on a payment plan?
Should I sell my car?—becomes a kind of blaring siren overriding
your internal monologue. You try to drink lukewarm water on
the side of your mouth with the fewest untreated cavities. Life
becomes a kind of self-destructive ultramarathon: How long
will I keep going? What's going to break next?

This kind of desperation drives a lot of horror stories. In his
book *America's Bitter Pill*,* Steven Brill famously profiled an elderly woman who had to work as a baggage handler to receive
the insurance she needed. Some kids, growing up uninsured
in poor families, are punished for going to the doctor because
their families can't afford the cost, and remain scared of doctors as adults. People who get injured on the job sometimes
turn to painkillers to keep them working so they and their
children don't lose the insurance tied to their job.

At some point, you just can't keep going. In 2009, 45,000 people
died from causes related to uninsurance.[16] 45,000 families. 45,000
entirely preventable deaths. These people should be alive—they
were *killed by* our health finance model. It has killed before, it has
killed hundreds of thousands of uninsured people since, and it
will kill again unless we drive a stake through its heart.

It is infinitely better to be insured than uninsured, but the
space between the two is much, much smaller than you might
hope. An increasing number of people who are insured and
poor, or insured and unable to use their insurance—sometimes called "underinsured"—face similar problems, the same
impossible choices, as uninsured people. There were 63 million underinsured adults in 2018, or a third of the adult population under 65.[17]

But not all insurances are alike. There are two basic categories of insurance in the United States: *public insurance* and

---

* *Bitter Pill* is a hell of a book because the first two-thirds really dissect several of
the structural problems in American insurance, and then the last third has the
stupidest conclusion ("Why not just have more private monopolies?") in print.

private insurance. Public insurance programs have been an essential means of promoting public health in America, and the ways they've been gutted for private profit offer fascinating, infuriating examples of how letting private companies hijack public services ends up wasting a lot of time and money for very little, if any, public benefit. Private insurance resembles the Blue Cross model from the 1920s: a private company takes your money and gives you some kind of insurance in exchange, while trying to make money for itself. Because this is a book about health justice, single-payer insurance, and the private insurance companies in the way, I will ultimately devote more of this section to the private sector than the public. But here is a quick description of how public insurance works today.

PUBLIC INSURANCE

Public insurance, or government-sponsored insurance, is an insurance model in which a government (or "public") agency is the primary payer of medical costs. Access to these government payers may be restricted by income, age, and other categories. It comes in a few major flavors: Medicare, Medicaid, and the Veterans Affairs (VA) healthcare administration.

Medicare

Medicare is an insurance program that is available to all people age 65 or older.* In 2017 it spent about $710 billion,[18] or a fifth of total national healthcare dollars. Its money comes almost

---

* You can also qualify for Medicare if you've had a disability and have received Social Security for two years, or if you have a permanent disability or end-stage renal disease.

entirely from the federal government. It was built slowly, over decades, and resembles less a continuous and whole object, or unified "Medicare," than a cluster of several noncontiguous subcomponents.

- **Medicare Part A** is free for people who receive Social Security payments; others need to pay a premium of approximately $420 a month.[19] (This means that if you were a stay-at-home parent or an unpaid family caregiver, you're paying a massive premium for Medicare.) Part A covers hospitalizations and emergency room charges. After a patient spends over $1,000 on hospital treatment and resulting care (like being transferred to a nursing facility), Medicare covers the bill in full for up to 60 days, then pushes those costs back onto the patient.
- **Medicare Part B** is a plan with a premium, or cost to join. It covers medical care outside emergency hospitalization— seeing a doctor, a specialist, etc. It costs a little under $150 a month. Then, after you spend about your first $200 at the doctor's office for the year, it covers 80 percent of the remaining bills you get from your doctor. The rest you pay out of pocket.
- Then there's **Medicare Part C**, aka Medicare Advantage, in which private insurance companies can offer private insurance plans to Medicare recipients. You pay the standard Medicare Part B premium, sometimes with an additional fee to the insurer. The federal government also pays the insurer a subsidy for insuring you. These plans bundle the services covered by Parts A, B, and D and— unlike Medicare—decrease or limit the money you spend out of pocket on healthcare. Medicare Advantage insurers also get money for special programs not available to normal Medicare—like government subsidies on Lyft rides

for patients who lack access to transit.* These plans are also usually very, very profitable for the insurance companies selling them—up to a 30 percent margin.[20] Of course, these companies like to protect those profits, and often do so by denying care to patients[21] or imposing restrictions on which doctors a patient can see or what care a patient can receive.

- **Medicare Part D** is another program you have to pay for to use. It covers drug costs, up to a point. If you need more than $3,750 of pharmaceutical drugs in a year, you're on the hook for 25 percent of your total drug costs.† Spend $5,000 in total drug costs, and Medicare kicks in again. You'll be charged 5 percent of your remaining drug bills. This might be fine if you need medicine for a short-term injury or infection, but it's quite a challenge for people with long-term conditions.‡

Let's review. Medicare Parts A and B are expensive programs with a lot of problems, plus they push costs onto the patient. Medicare Part C, the private option, is exempt from those requirements, plus gets federal money to invest in new accessory

---

* This is of course an incredible scam, but it's also far from optimal for patients. Lyft is not a medical transport service. Patients are stuck sharing rides with other people, getting stuck in traffic, or riding in vehicles or with drivers ill equipped for their healthcare needs: https://www.forbes.com/sites/bruce-japsen/2018/04/08/for-uber-and-lyft-medicare-could-be-the-next-profitable-ride/#da01b571b0f5.

† This used to be a much worse situation, in which someone who needed drugs would have to pay for them all out of pocket in this coverage gap—known as the "donut hole"—but it is scheduled to be closed in 2019.

‡ Those with multiple chronic conditions are more likely to hit the donut hole. See: Yuting Zhang, et al. "The Effects Of The Coverage Gap On Drug Spending: A Closer Look At Medicare Part D," *Health Affairs*, March/April 2009, available at: https://www.healthaffairs.org/doi/full/10.1377/hlthaff.28.2.w317.

benefits or incentives. Does something seem strange to you? Why do private plans get these abilities when the public ones don't? There's no reason Medicare couldn't restrict or limit out-of-pocket spending for its patients. Why would the private plans, which receive both your money and a government handout, be singularly able to restrict out-of-pocket spending and be extremely profitable to the private company selling them? Why have we given private plans, which we subsidize with public money, these abilities the public plans don't get? Does it seem like, maybe, the standard Medicare plans have been hollowed out or made weak so that Part C seems like the most appealing option? Part C has represented an increasing share of American medical costs over the past few years, even though it's a woefully inefficient use of government money.[22] You might even suspect that the relative weakness of Parts A and B is intentionally designed to drive people into the privatized Part C option. I do!

Medicare Advantage—privatized Medicare—represents the government weakening its own insurance programs so it can waste money on paying private companies to do a worse and more expensive job of insuring people. But I don't want to dwell too long on Medicare Advantage plans. Suffice it to say, they are very profitable, they receive a lot of extra money from the federal government, and even the executives of Medicare Advantage companies have started whistle-blowing[23] about— in their terms—the grift they're getting away with.

Which is a disappointment, because Medicare has one of the largest advantages of any actor in American healthcare: size. Medicare insures about 44 million people, or 15 percent of the nation's population. It is, by *far*, the largest insurer in the United States. It uses that size to do a lot of pretty cool things. For example, most private insurance companies every year have to renegotiate how much they'll pay for various procedures and medicines. Since, in most places, insurers need the hospital more than the hospital needs the insurer,* insurers are forced to accept inflated prices for care (which they then just pass back to their customers). That's not the case with Medicare. Every year, Medicare determines how much it will pay for services. Hospitals can decide to reject those prices, but then they can't accept Medicare, which means turning away 44 million customers with guaranteed payment. As a result, the vast majority of hospitals and most providers accept Medicare patients.†

This kind of structure—access to a massive pile of money, but only if you adopt certain requirements—is the model by which hospitals in America were formally integrated. Segregated hospitals in the South were told they would not be eligible to receive Medicare funds unless they admitted patients of all races. Though they resisted, at the zero hour they caved.‡ It's amazing what you can do with an economy of scale! Behold, the power of Medicare!

---

* Think about it like this: suppose you're an insurance company in a city with one or two dominant hospital chains. If you don't come to an agreement with a major hospital, you won't cover your customers' care there. People generally are unhappy about simultaneously paying out the ass for insurance and not being able to go to the emergency room nearest them, and therefore won't buy your insurance plan. (This presumes that the customer is able to determine which hospitals are "in" and "out of network," or where they can go to get their care covered and where they cannot. That a person can do this is a necessary corporate fantasy for the continuation of the private insurance industry.)

† Nine out of ten primary care physicians take Medicare patients, per Kaiser: https://www.kff.org/medicare/issue-brief/primary-care-physicians-accepting-medicare-a-snapshot/.

‡ Much of the credit for this goes to the tireless volunteer armies of hospital investigators and caseworkers. For a wonderful documentary on this, check out *The Power to Heal: Medicare and the Civil Rights Revolution.*

Medicaid

Medicaid is both a state and federally funded program. In wealthier states, like California, both state and federal governments split the cost equally. In poorer states, like Mississippi, the federal government contributes up to 75 percent of the total budget. The federal government sets standards for care and what needs must be met, but the states are free to develop their own programs and administer them as they see fit.

Approximately 66 million people enrolled in Medicaid in 2018. Since it is a program paid for by 52 different actors (50 states, the District of Columbia, and the federal government) it does not have the same singular economy of scale Medicare enjoys. It does, however, have the privilege of offering a discounted rate from Medicare.* Approximately 70 percent of physicians accept Medicaid, but this number (and the cost discount) varies dramatically from state to state.[24]

Unlike Medicare, which is available to anyone older than 65, states have a lot of discretion over determining who's eligible for Medicaid. Generally speaking, poorer people have more healthcare needs (we talked about this earlier and we'll talk more about this later). As a result, many states claim that Medicaid is too expensive for them to afford, and thus impose aggressive restrictions on who could use the program. For example, Texas restricts Medicaid eligibility to:

- people with disabilities;
- parents (and *only* parents) who make less than $3,600 a year;

---

* This leads some hospitals to complain that they can't afford to see Medicaid patients, which is occasionally true but often rings flat in the face of multi-million-dollar executive salaries and capital expenditures on luxury hospital accommodations.

- low-income pregnant people (household income less than $24,000 if they're single); and
- children whose families have a household income less than twice the poverty level (but not the families themselves).

Clunky, isn't it? Cruel, too. This means that, for example, if you're a Texan who's "just" poor (maybe you're a pizza delivery driver, a bartender, a nanny, or all three)* or a single parent who makes more than $300 a month, you're ineligible for Medicaid. Rough!

Medicaid expansion under the ACA became a voluntary process, and state Medicaid programs have significant leeway to determine what they do and do not cover. As a result, Medicaid programs vary widely in both their eligibility criteria as well as their benefits. Nowhere is this more apparent than in the case of long-term care (LTC) and home and community-based services (HCBS). Long-term care is the kind of care that Steve, from the introduction of the book, needs. When he gets paid help at home, whether from Kyle, his mother, or an outside caregiver, that's an example of HCBS, and a kind of long-term care.

Long-term care in America is generally hidden out of sight. When people with disabilities are unable to take care of themselves without assistance, they are pushed into corporate nursing homes rampant with grift, abuse, and corruption in the pursuit of profit. Lawmakers in Arkansas and Kentucky have been caught working with nursing home corporations to make it harder for patients to sue for malpractice. Trapped, unable to live freely, work, or leave: for people with disabilities, nursing homes are, frankly, equal part warehouse and hospice.

---

* Nobody should be denied the liberty of healthcare, end of sentence. But of all the people to prohibit basic, cheap healthcare, it's particularly absurd that we've chosen the people who take care of our children, handle our food, and serve us drinks!

Even if Medicaid offers HCBS, its means-testing restrictions can be brutal and oppressive. Disabled couples with too much money in the bank—$22,000 in New York, plus a max of $1,233 in monthly income—often need to spend down or divorce to qualify. Sometimes you have cases like Steve's from the introduction, where he can't make more than $2,000 in a year. This is because Medicaid wants to make sure that people who use HCBS are really, *really* poor.

Medicaid is a paradox, in that it's arguably the most important (and a very cost-efficient) healthcare program in the United States, but it's also under constant assault in both nominally liberal and conservative states. Since it is administered independently by each state, it is home to the most "innovation" in American healthcare—both in finding ways to help more people more proactively, and also in finding ways to restrict access to care, or punish people for being sick. If you want to find a program that explores how to provide comprehensive social services and advocacy for poor pregnant people, you can find it in Medicaid (for example, the Strong Start programs). If you want to find a way to punish those pregnant people after they give birth by removing their right to privacy and demanding continual checkups, check-ins, and surveillance as a requirement for care, you can also find it in Medicaid. In some states Medicaid is entirely privatized, contracted out to "managed care" companies that restrict provider access and put patients through endless denials, appeal processes, and hassle—while rapidly increasing state Medicaid spending and, conveniently, turning a profit. Medicaid is a program exhilarating in its effectiveness and its empathy; it is a program devastating in its cruelty and coldness.

There is a lesson to be learned here: given the chance to accept a huge amount of federal money to help people, some elected officials will reject it outright for political or ideological reasons. Given the opportunity to wield denial and neglect like a cudgel, some officials will choose to do so, even at the expense of their own state or agency. A just healthcare model can make no room for the few powerful people who seek to be bullies, to use healthcare to harm the vulnerable.

A Brief Note on Work Requirements

Any discussion of Medicaid requires a discussion of **Medicaid waivers**. States can petition the Department of Health and Human Services to be released from some of the requirements of the Medicaid program, for purposes of "experimentation," under Section 1115 of the Social Security Act. It's an extremely cool statute that lets states have more local control over how they spend their healthcare dollars, with the explicit goal of expanding coverage while reducing cost.* This means that a regional agency more finely attuned to the particular needs of its population can use Medicaid money to invest in the things its population needs—like specific community outreach, housing, or transportation programs. Neat.

Except, like all policy, it is vulnerable to bad actors. There is a rising movement to use Section 1115 waivers to shrink Medicaid programs or push out "undeserving" populations—efforts that disproportionately affect poor people and people of color.† The most visible focus of these waivers is "work requirements."

The Republican work requirements movement claims that there is some mass of Medicaid recipients who are "getting away" with "free handouts" from the government, and out of an impulse toward "fiscal responsibility,"

---

*   Prior to Medicaid expansion under the ACA, states used Medicaid waivers to expand coverage to childless adults: https://www.kff.org/report-section/section-1115-medicaid-demonstration-waivers-issue-brief/.

†   This might remind you of the poorhouse movements of the 1800s.

they must be "encouraged to work" by making sure everyone who receives Medicaid is forced to get a job.*

This is categorically wrong. This does not "encourage" anyone to work. Virtually everyone who receives Medicaid already works if they are able.[†][‡] What this *does* do is force people to endure long waits[25] or use websites that don't work (plus, many Medicaid recipients don't have reliable access to the Internet)[26] to log their hours with a severely understaffed benefits office. The offices aren't helped by these waivers either: the work requirements waiver in Tennessee, for example, included no funding to help staff or upgrade the department that would now have to verify employment for 1.5 million people every month, a task with which it struggles greatly.

These seem like a series of managerial blunders, the side effects of bumbling bureaucrats or pointy-haired *Dilbert* bosses, but they're not. This is all *intentional*. The plan isn't "financial responsibility" or "encouraging people to work." The plan is punishment. Punishment of poor people, punishment of people of color, and punishment of sick people, the "undeserving" poor—a theme we will return to in this book. We are told we are being made to suffer the "lazy moocher" who dwells at the bottom of the safety net, taking all our money. We are

---

*   You might recognize this from when the Clintons did literally the same thing at the federal level as they cut Temporary Assistance for Needy Families (TANF).

†   Or, like Steve from the introduction, are restricted from working by income restrictions. They get you both ways. See also https://www.kff.org/medicaid /issue-brief/implications-of-work-requirements-in-medicaid-what-does-the -data-say/. ("Most Medicaid enrollees who can work are already working but could face barriers in complying with reporting requirements. More than six in ten adult enrollees are working.")

‡   And if they don't, who cares? There's nothing moral about working or not working.

told that we must *punish* them, because Work is Good.*
These waivers exist to bully vulnerable people; to make
them wait in forever-long lines, in offices with neither
the space, funding, or even *basic technology* to verify their
employment; and then deny them healthcare. It is very
literally murderous.†

Veterans Affairs (VA)

A third model of public insurance is the Veterans Affairs program. The VA is a medical provider owned by the public that
treats a subsection of American military members and veterans—often an older, sicker population. Eligible veterans go to
the VA for care and are billed based on their income and whether
they have a service-related disability or condition. Single people
making less than $32,000 a year usually pay nothing. Other peo-
ple who use the VA often still enroll in private insurance plans
to cover these co-pay costs—similar to Medicare Part C.‡

About 9 million people are enrolled in the VA system, and
VA facilities train the highest number of doctors in the United
States.[27] However, the VA is being hamstrung by a growing
number of enrollees combined with insufficient funding.
While the VA's budget is slightly less subject to the political

---

*   It's fine. Work is fine.

†   Means-testing literally has its origins in the early eugenics movement. It is an
attempt to determine who is worthy of aid from the state and who is not. It draws
inspiration from early British efforts to determine which colonized people were
mentally inferior and therefore unable of being saved or alleviated and, therefore,
whose receipt of assistance would be a waste. Contrast this with discussions
around the "culture of poverty," a common argument against giving poor people
of color welfare benefits.

‡   "If we can find a way to make private companies profit, we'll do it, no matter
who suffers!"

footballing of Congress than other healthcare provisions, funding is still critically below what it would need to be to treat all veterans who were promised care upon completion of their stints as soldiers.[28] The number of aging Vietnam veterans and people wounded during our perpetual invasions in the Middle East, combined with pending legislation that would let more people exposed to Agent Orange qualify for VA care,[29] mean the VA is often "at capacity." As a result, members of the VA are triaged (e.g., people with "50 percent disability" are seen ahead of "people with 10 percent" disability; people with less money are seen before people with more money; people with Medals of Honor are given priority over undecorated veterans), which results in angry patients, political stress, and death—a 2015 study showed that wait times might have contributed to the death of 307,000 vets waiting for VA healthcare.[30]

There's a simple answer to the problem of increased demand and restricted capacity: spend more money to expand capacity. But exploiting this friction is a VA privatization movement, which alleges that the problems faced by the VA can only be resolved by private companies. The proponents of VA privatization are not troubled by the fact that these private companies are notorious in virtually every other sector of healthcare for costing more while squeezing money from and restricting care for those who are most vulnerable. They simply don't work; but that's not the goal. The goal of this privatization movement is, of course, the same as any other movement for reactionary austerity. It seeks to starve a program of its budget and use its resulting weakness to justify forking over work to rich people and their private companies, badly, for profit.

There is also a separate military hospital system for people currently employed by the armed forces. For their spouses and children, a program called TRICARE exists—a privately administered insurance program paid for by the military, which uses private doctors and private hospitals.

Indian Health Service (IHS)

Lastly, there is the Indian Health Service (IHS), which treats Native Americans. Unlike Medicare and Medicaid, which are funded through the Social Security Act, IHS is funded through an appropriation of the Department of the Interior. Its chronically and critically low funding, combined with the social and structural harms inflicted upon Native reservations, cause deep problems for IHS. I want to analyze those social and structural problems later in this book, so we will revisit the IHS in Part 3.

★   ★   ★

At their best, these public insurers are vehicles for using public money—your money—to provide care to your family, your friends, and your community. When they are ripped off, you are ripped off. When they are made inadequate, your grandparents and your children suffer. And they are, very much, being ripped off and made inadequate. So whether you're covered by Medicare or Medicaid or the VA or not, your skin is already in the game with American public insurance.

PRIVATE INSURANCE

But not all people in the United States use public insurance. Most of us are being bounced around the American **private insurance system** (or have no insurance at all).[31] It is a heinous machine that causes agony and pain for the profit and pleasure of the millionaires and billionaires who own it. Let's investigate that system from the bottom up.

The smallest—and, despite what the insurance companies

insist, the most important—component of private insurance is the **person**. You, me, and everyone we know. Generally speaking, most of us probably won't have major healthcare spending this year. But if we have an accident or emergency, if we ever need surgery, or if we have or develop a chronic health condition like asthma or schizophrenia or cystic fibrosis, we'd be on the hook for up to hundreds of thousands of dollars—sometimes *millions* of dollars—of hospital bills and other medical costs. We don't want to do that, so if we're lucky enough to be able to afford it, we purchase insurance to help mitigate these staggering costs.

We can get insurance in one of two ways: either by purchasing a plan directly from the insurer on the "individual insurance market," or through our employers. Employer-sponsored insurance comes in two modes. The first is traditional insurance, in which the employer buys plans operated entirely by a third-party insurance company, and in which the insurance risk is spread across all people on the insurer's plans, even if those people work at many different companies. The other is a self-insured plan, in which the employer pools all the risk among only its own employees, though it may still contract out a third party to administer the insurance. Whatever the avenue, the contract being purchased is called an *insurance plan*.

Insurance plans are agreements between people (now *customers*) and insurance companies. We pay the insurance company a fixed amount of money (called a *premium*, and usually billed monthly) in exchange for two things. If we go to a doctor, a facility, or a hospital the insurance company has a business relationship with (or that is *in network*), the insurance company will both negotiate down the bill the doctor or hospital charges, and, ideally, cover the cost.[*]

---

[*] This presumes that all the doctors you see at that hospital are covered by the plan, which is often not the case. In Texas, for example, there's a particular problem with anesthesiologists, who refuse to join insurance plans, even at

But, of course, insurance companies don't always pick up the check. The insurance plan usually contains two additional items:

- The *co-pay*, the amount you must pay to see a doctor covered by your network. This can be a percentage or a fixed amount (e.g., "50 percent of bill," "$50 to see a primary care provider," or "$500 to visit the emergency room").
- The *deductible*, or an amount you must spend in a year on healthcare *before* the insurance company starts covering the rest. If your insurance plan has a deductible of $5,000, the insurance company starts picking up the check after you've spent $5,000 out of your own money on healthcare costs "in the field." Your premium doesn't count toward the deductible. It's considered to be more of a "membership fee" rather than a healthcare cost.

If you want a plan with a low co-pay and low deductible (usually because you're sick and need to use your insurance plan a lot), it's going to cost you a much higher premium. The opposite is true: if you can only afford a low premium, it's going to cost you a lot more to use your insurance plan.* This is only for "medical" care—things like vision care and dental care have their own insurance plans and their own insurance companies.†

There are also categories of insurance plans—HMO, PPO, EPO, and POS. It's a dizzying list of initialisms, or America's

---

hospitals that do, and who therefore can charge patients more for services they're unable to decline.

* For reference: in one NYC insurer's plans for 2019: I, a 30-year-old man, can pick plans starting at a $480/month premium and $4,000 deductible up to a $1,000/month premium with a $0 deductible. I can afford neither of these, but I also have significant monthly medical expenses. Don't you love the free market?

† Dental care and vision care are obviously components of medical care; but, again, this thing doesn't make sense.

least exciting pinball high-score screen. To make it very simple: insurance companies make more money if they control where and how you seek healthcare. Part of this makes sense: if you see five doctors, and none of them talk to each other, you could receive redundant or even harmful care. This is a problem that we could solve by having easily portable personal medical records (or even a federal database of medical records). Instead, the insurer smells an opportunity to profit by "coordinating care," and butts in. Sometimes it compels you to get referrals from a designated primary care provider (PCP) before you can see any kind of specialist, and if you don't, it's not covered (this is the "health maintenance organization," or HMO, model). Sometimes you're allowed to see doctors without prior permission, but if they're not in network, you're saddled with the cost (the "preferred provider organization," or PPO, model). The other ones are weird hybrids of the two.

This stuff is pretty complicated, and most of it doesn't make sense to people who need healthcare—ultimately, I think, because this isn't a system designed for their benefit. Thinking about it just makes me want to chip my own teeth. If you're confused, perhaps you'll find solace when I remind you that this is not an intentionally designed system: it is one that emerged like a prehistoric corpse from an ancient and foul bog, and is now stinking up the place.

The owner of an insurance plan is the **insurer**. Insurers are organizations, usually private companies, who make money by selling insurance plans and receiving subsidies from public money.* Insurers sell as many insurance plans as possible to customers in exchange for premiums. These premiums—plus the government subsidies—are pooled and used to pay some of the healthcare costs of customers, as

---

* Many insurance companies see themselves as financial companies as well as healthcare companies.

well as the company's various corporate expenses, like pay-roll, advertising, and rent; and then the rest is kept as profit. Since most people who can afford insurance don't spend much money on healthcare in a year—again, remember that 5 percent of people drive half of all costs—that pool of money (called a "risk pool" because it *pools* the collective *risk* that any given customer will be expensive across a large number of typically inexpensive customers—kind of like the opposite of an office lottery pool) usually contains quite a bit of profit for the insurance company.[32] In fact, insurers are accustomed to making *so much* profit that the ACA enforced laws compelling insurers to use at least 85 percent of their revenue on paying out insurance claims (the "medical loss ratio") instead of spending it on itself or pocketing it.

Each of these kinds of insurance—Medicare, Medicaid, and the other kinds of public insurance, plus the various private insurers—is sometimes known as a "payer," because they're (often) the organizations that pay healthcare costs. Because there are multiple payers, and multiple kinds of payers, America's healthcare system is described as a **multi-payer system**.

Okay. Does this all make sense? Well, no, it doesn't. But hopefully now you see the basic contours of how insurance works. Now let's talk about something truly stupefying: the fact that *when you use your insurance plan, your insurer loses money*.

THE PERVERSE RELATIONSHIP BETWEEN YOU AND YOUR INSURER

This might sound like an oversimplification—your insurance company loses money every time you go to the doctor—but it's very much at the root of why you feel pinched in the gears of American health insurance. Private insurance companies don't have the same kind of scale that Medicare, or even a state Medicaid plan, has.* To compensate, it taps into the sub-industry of predicting how many people on a plan will actually use their insurance given a particular arrangement of the variables within an insurer's control. That is to say: "For a certain combination of premium, co-pay, and deductible, how many other people are likely to go see the doctor? Will they see the doctor often enough that we lose money? How many people with chronic conditions will buy our insurance plan? How do we make sure we lose as little money on them as possible?"

This is a wicked algebra, but it's all the insurer can do if it wants to appease its shareholders or owners.† Because the alternative is catastrophic to the insurance company: if they attract too many people who *use* their insurance plans to see the doctor; if too many people with chronic conditions sign up (for example, a person with hemophilia, whose care can cost up to a million dollars a year); if they can't draw customers who *won't* use their insurance plans (either because they don't need to or can't afford to), the insurer's per-person costs skyrocket.

When an insurance company's per-person costs increase, it compensates by increasing premiums. When premiums increase, people who can't afford those premiums drop out.‡ So far, this sucks, but it makes sense, right? We've pretended healthcare is a normal market good.

---

* Even though the aggregated Blue Cross Blue Shield companies insure a collective 100 million people, there are many regions within each state that operate as different insurance markets, with different providers to negotiate with and different local needs.

† Won't somebody please think of the shareholders?

‡ This presumes that there's either another plan on the market at a lower cost, or that people aren't mandated to purchase insurance (or the penalty for breaking the mandate is insufficient).

Except. People who are sick, people who are expensive to insure—they can't *afford* to drop out of their insurance plan. How else would they be able to afford the care that keeps them alive? And if they change plans, they might not be able to see their doctor. Coerced into the annual indignation of rising costs, they grit their teeth and hang on for as long as they can. And by this determination, they once again increase the per-person costs of the insurer. Next year, premiums will increase to compensate. The cycle continues.

Thus, the dream of a private insurer is a large and uneventful customer base. A risk-less risk pool. A million customers who pay their premiums every month and who never get hepatitis or get into car accidents or get other expensive conditions. But this corporate-utopian vision doesn't reflect the way illness works: there are simply always going to be a bunch of people who get sick or who need expensive care. Because the insurer doesn't have the ability to make sick people *well*, or to prevent illness or accidents in its customers, and absent the ability to just imagine away the customers who cause most of the medical costs, all the private insurer can do is find ways to kick out sick customers, or coerce them into leaving.

Private insurers are very good at this. They drop coverage for drugs sick people need; they end contracts with doctors and specialists who treat the sickest patients (and are therefore the doctors costing the most money to the insurance company).* In Florida and Illinois, insurance companies are being sued for making it intentionally difficult, complicated, and expensive for people with HIV/AIDS to get the drugs

---

* It is also true that there are "bad apple" or "low-quality" providers who cost some amount of money per patient that the insurer determines is excessive—for example, someone who orders what the insurer would determine to be unnecessary MRIs. But purging doctors like this is a heavy-handed approach to cost savings, and one that implicitly ignores patient agency. A sick person should not be the battlefield between an insurer and a doctor.

they need.[33] This is done, the suit alleges, so that these people with diseases will just give up and go to other insurance companies.

Or there's mental health coverage, something insurance companies across the country have worked hard to deny their customers. Because mental disorders and mental illness* can be managed but not cured, and often include hospitalizations or other expensive episodes of acute care,[†] it's not very profitable to cover the people who have them. If you were to give them cheap and accessible mental healthcare, the logic goes, they'll use it, and you will have to pay for it, and that doesn't make shareholders very happy. Insurer discrimination against mental healthcare became so bad that even rich people complained about it, as former House Representative Patrick Kennedy published an essay on the phenomenon.[34] The battle to avoid selling insurance to the mentally unwell is waged on fronts beyond consumer relations. One of the reasons it's very difficult to find a mental health provider, for example, is because insurance companies tend to offer very low reimbursements for providing mental healthcare.[‡] As a result, many mental health providers don't—or can't, or won't—accept insurance. It's a particularly rotten scheme.

It turns out that because insurance companies lose money when you get sick, the task of an insurance company is to

---

*   Mental illnesses like depression, ADHD, and schizophrenia are just as much physical as illnesses like the flu or pneumonia—they're just less visible and thus easier to discriminate against.

†   "Acute care" refers to urgent, short-term care, like going to the ER for a lawn-mower accident or going to an urgent care center for an asthma attack. It is contrasted against "long-term" or "chronic" care, which includes things like hospice care and dialysis treatments for kidney failure.

‡   There's a relatively new class-action lawsuit about this, this time with a new wrinkle—alleging that giant insurer UnitedHealth underpays for mental health work done by anyone other than a doctor: https://www.classaction. org/media/smith-v-united-healthcare-insurance-company-et-al.pdf.

make sick people, as much as it can, someone else's problem. Before the Affordable Care Act was passed, people who didn't get insurance from their job and who thus needed individual insurance had to apply directly to insurance companies to purchase insurance plans. These applications included huge, invasive surveys detailing every aspect of their life. If they were deemed to be a risky customer—that is, if they were someone who was sick or who needed expensive care or who had a history of severe illness—their application would be denied. (These are the "preexisting conditions" you may have heard about in the news.) This is an ideal outcome for the insurance industry: hang on to us for as long as we're profitable, then throw us away; let us bounce from company to company like a pinball, until we're no longer able to pay our hundreds or thousands of dollars to the multibillion-dollar insurance companies,* until we fall and are lost, abandoned, until we lose everything and pray we qualify for meager government care.

★　★　★

This is what we mean when we say we live in a world in which healthcare is a *commodity* like bananas or oil or wheat. Futures on your heart, your lungs, your chance of getting diabetes, whether your mom's glaucoma gets worse before she turns 65 and goes on Medicare, are fiddled with and speculated about and, ultimately, bought and sold for profit by private companies. We're just portable, unstable profit pods, utterly dependent upon the insurer that drains us.

Except, unlike oil or wheat, we don't have a commodity relationship with our own *health*. For one, we're very cost in-

---

* The nation's top six health insurance companies made $6 billion in the second quarter of 2017, all while the ACA was dangling on the edge of a knife in Congress: https://www.cnbc.com/2017/08/05/top-health-insurers-profit-surge-29-percent-to-6-billion-dollars.html.

elastic: if we are in pain, or if our kids are in pain, once we're in the hospital, we tend to do whatever our doctor says we should do.* Unlike beer or wrestling pay-per-views, we can't really "buy less" of healthcare in any meaningful way—we either buy it when we need it, or we go without.† So we go without. And then we need more—much more—later.

It's awful. It's all a scam. It's a scam that has killed millions of people in America and will kill millions more. It's a lie that holds sick people, people with disabilities, and their families for ransom, and then throws them to the wolves once there's no more profit to be drained. All the while, the insurance company looks at us with wide eyes. *Well, gosh*, it says. *We'd really love to help. But it's just too expensive for us. It's really unfair, but some people just don't get to afford healthcare. Something should be done, but we can't do it.*‡

This is the great and wicked trick that has been played on us. We've been browbeaten into viewing healthcare as a *transaction* between a customer and an insurance company, or an insurance company and a hospital, instead of a relationship between a person, their body, their community, and their doctor. That's perverted. *We have mistaken the profit motives of companies for healthcare.*

And over time, we've delegated the responsibility of providing this insurance to employers.

This is pretty hosed, because it results in a status of total employer domination. Your access to things like blood transfusions, contraception, or hormone therapy is determined by

---

* That's literally what a doctor's job is.

† There are of course people who do things like buy their medications from Mexico or India, which is a valiant effort to protect oneself against overwhelming cost, and an entirely reasonable thing to do—just not a scalable one.

‡ The preferred solutions offered by insurance companies usually involve either the federal government paying insurance companies a lot of money to insure people, or the federal government insuring the unprofitable people itself.

the whims of your employer. Don't like your employer? Have a shitty job with shitty working conditions? Insurance means you have to stay.

You're kind of screwed over three ways here: One, employers have the ability to determine what services the insurance they offer covers. Two, self-insured companies can claim exemption from covering things like abortion or contraception for faith-based reasons. Three, so can hospitals: 38 percent of women[*] of reproductive age live in a county with no abortion provider.[*]

But maybe you aren't lucky enough to have an employer, or maybe your employer is an asshole[†] who decides you need to grovel before he'll offer you the privilege of forking over more than you pay in rent for a shitty insurance plan. Maybe your employer cuts your hours just below the threshold where he's legally required to offer you insurance. Maybe overtime means you make too much to qualify for public insurance, but you can't afford the employer's insurance plan. Then you're just left behind.

Christ, what a mess. The people who profit from the commodification of our bodies have decided that it is acceptable to shackle the well-being of children to whether or not their parents have a good job—or if they were lucky enough to have gone back in time 40 years, learned to code,[‡] and found a benevolent employer.[§]

This is insurance. This is hell. Welcome to the hell world of America 2019.

---

[*]   https://onlinelibrary.wiley.com/doi/full/10.1363/46e0414 ("Women" is the language of the survey.)

[†]   The Street Fight Radio podcast's "Small Business Tyrants" series is my favorite repository of these people.

[‡]   The idiotic, cruel "miners should learn to code!" movement, blessedly short-lived, never seemed to reckon with the fact that there are very few front-end development jobs in coal country.

[§]   And sometimes not even then. I met a man, a construction worker, whose employer offered a high-deductible plan—and offered to cover his family only if he remained employed for three years.

COST

It gets worse.* The costs of healthcare keep increasing. They increase *much* faster than inflation—almost 25 percent faster since 2007.[35] They've been increasing since we first began recording them back in the late nineteenth century. Let's examine why, and who's doing it.

Some of these cost increases happen for good reasons. The quality of care you can receive in the United States, if you can afford it, is much stronger than it was a few decades ago. Far fewer people die from diseases like smallpox or malaria than at the turn of the twentieth century, and emergencies like heart attacks and trauma are far less of an immediate death sentence than they were even two or three generations ago.† So we spent more money helping more people live longer and healthier lives. That's a fantastic use of money.

But this isn't the underlying explanation for cost increases. You can represent healthcare spending with an (overly) simple formula:

Healthcare spending = healthcare prices x usage

"Usage," or "utilization" in health policy lingo, just means "how often healthcare services are used." So are American healthcare costs increasing because of higher prices, are people going to the doctor more often, or both?

The answer is, unequivocally, higher prices. *The costs are*

---

* Of course it gets worse. We're *way* too early in this book for things not to get worse.

† In the United States, that is. This is not the case in many other countries around the world, and this is an injustice the United States has contributed to, and benefitted from, through its tireless colonial plundering of other countries' natural and economic resources.

high because the prices are high. This is such a simple and repeatedly proven fact, and it's also very quickly ignored in the pursuit of private profit. People in the United States tend to use fewer hospital and physician services ("less utilization") but get more specialized surgeries like knee replacements and C-sections than people in other countries with lower per-person costs.[36] Medical care is getting better,[*] but specialized medical technology for specialty patients is not skewing the American cost curve so much higher than other countries'. Rather, providers and manufacturers are selling all goods and services of American healthcare, specialized and not, at greatly inflated and greatly increasing unit costs.

So despite what your insurance company might want you to believe, these cost increases aren't occurring just because we're bad at going to the doctor the "right" amount. Most of these cost increases occur because hospital CEOs, pharmaceutical companies, and device manufacturers keep finding more and more ways to charge more money for the same procedures, or ways to rack up fees for unnecessary services, and no private insurer can stop them.

SOME WONDERFUL EXAMPLES OF BLOATED COSTS

However much grift you think there is in healthcare spending—multiply it by ten, then ten, then ten once more. There is a whole vast and wicked ocean of healthcare-related corporations that, like every other company on earth, spend a lot of money finding ways to make more money. They are very effective at this. They have created a strange market for the "commodity"

---

[*]   Well, for people who can afford it. Plus, there's the specter of provider-induced demand; for example, many pregnant people report being pressured into getting a C-section, and many C-sections are unnecessarily, and expensively, performed.

of healthcare where there are no stable or fixed prices, where providers sell as many services as possible regardless of need, and where new competitors in a market ultimately *increase* the costs felt by patients. It hits us from several angles: we suffer the brunt of increased healthcare premiums; we feel anxiety as our state governments claim they can't invest in infrastructure or other necessities because of the costs of Medicaid; we watch Congress whine that it can't pay for Medicare.*

An underlying principle of American healthcare costs is that all prices are fake. There is no rational accountancy science summing up line items to determine how much a healthcare service costs. There is no consistency. The goal is, explicitly, to charge as much as is possible to be paid.

My favorite example of healthcare costs being driven by healthcare prices is in the MRI (magnetic resonance imaging) machine. You're probably acquainted with MRIs as the cool tubes that perform very comprehensive scans of your body parts and brain. You may also know of them as giant machines that print money.

They print so much money, in fact, that the average MRI scan in the United States costs *five times more* than a scan from the same machine, performing the same procedure, when located in Australia.[37] But you don't need to go so far from home to get that kind of wild disparity. In a 2013 survey, former *Washington Post* reporter Sarah Kliff worked with healthcare data company Castlight† to find that MRI prices in the metro D.C. area ranged from $400 to $2,183 across hospitals: same procedure, same machine, another fivefold disparity.[38]

---

* It's almost trite to point out that this complaint is never raised about funding endless war or massive corporate tax breaks and other subsidies.

† I think this is what they do? Castlight appears to have at one point been a pricing transparency company (cool!), but now their website says things like "Integrate. Personalize. Guide. Engage," which I can't translate. Guess medical pricing is too hard for the innovations of the private sector.

It gets wilder than that. A single hospital, using the literal same MRI machine, in the same month, will vary its prices for scans by that machine from person to person, most often because the hospital changes the amount it charges based upon the contract it has with the patient's insurer. This happens so frequently that this kind of same-device, same-service, different-price discrepancy is responsible for up to one-fifth of *all* pricing discrepancies in the United States.[39]

So. Who do we blame for this mess of runaway healthcare costs? Are they just the natural equivocations of the market? No—healthcare costs spring up *so* eagerly, *much* faster than inflation, a rate and consequence unmatched by any other sector. Is it just "the way things are"? No—while every country faces down growing healthcare costs, their meteoric rise is singularly American. So who is doing this to us?

There is a school of thought that lays the blame for healthcare costs at the feet of the people who need healthcare. (They seek it "irresponsibly," we're told.) This is a callous argument advanced by smart people whose livelihoods depend on them pretending not to know better.

To the patient—even to the overly prepared patient, with PDFs of insurance plans and WebMD printouts at hand—American healthcare is a vast and incomprehensible maze, obscene in design and fatal in consequence. Its every navigation—will there be an opening at the clinic? Will my insurance cover this? For the services for which my insurance will inevitably skimp, can I afford the cost?—requires a small mystery of faith.

To blame this patient for going to the "wrong" hospital, seeing the "wrong" doctor, or waiting too long to get care is to blame the Athenian prisoner for being trampled by the Minotaur. It is never the patients' fault that their healthcare system is designed to harm them.

Instead, it may not surprise you to learn that rising costs

come from a constellation of American corporations exploiting every loophole and unregulated lever available to them to make as much profit as possible at the expense of patients' long-term well-being. Often, they do this while receiving hefty subsidies from public money (or while receiving exemptions from paying taxes). Healthcare costs in America are driven up by dozens of actors, each of which acts in ways that increase cost for others, who in turn act in ways that increase costs back at them. It's a circular firing squad, and nobody involved will change of their own accord. While virtually every company in the "healthcare" industry is responsible for increased costs—including insurers—I'm going to focus here on three examples from the *provider* side: equipment manufacturers, pharmaceutical companies, and big corporate hospitals.

Equipment Manufacturers

Equipment manufacturers are corporations that manufacture, sell, and sometimes resell durable medical equipment (DME)—everything from tongue depressors to hearing aids to pacemakers. They invent a lot of interesting and essential new devices—and they also use their elaborate sales systems to push a lot of junk into hospitals, and we pay for it.

When bringing new devices to market, device manufacturers benefit from a particularly jarring loophole—the 510(k) program—in getting FDA approval: if the item to be sold is categorized somewhere between the trivial (like a cotton ball) and the "life-threatening or life-sustaining," the device manufacturer can apply for an exemption from clinical trials by claiming it is "substantially equivalent" to a device already on the market. A company just needs to say "this is basically the same thing as a device that already exists," and through 510(k), as recently as 2015, they have an 85 percent chance of being cleared for the market.[40] The only problem is that these devices—which aren't carefully checked to see if they work, or at least don't break—have a funny habit of being less safe when used in practice. A health researcher testifying at an FDA hearing about the program reported that "from 2005 to 2009, 70 percent of high-risk-device recalls involved products that had gone to market through the 510(k) program."*

Why do hospitals buy these failing devices? Because device manufacturers deploy large, and persistent, sales forces. In *An American Sickness,* Elisabeth Rosenthal describes this relationship between device manufacturers and hospitals:

> Device makers start courting young orthopedists during their residencies and fellowships . . . because doctors get accustomed to the products they learn on . . .
>
> They formed alliances with doctors they considered "influencers." . . . With the 510(k) programs, device makers could readily reward the surgeons with patents and profits or funding for pet research projects . . .
>
> Part of the sales deal is that the [device maker] reps typically serve as unpaid assistants in the OR, helping surgeons install the devices they sell, a new tool at the ready to adjust a knee implant, for example. It was free help, and the good reps made operations go more smoothly . . .
>
> With the device makers' clever business models, such assistance was rendered almost essential because each implant is installed with brand-specific screws and tools, and often even on a brand-specific operating table.[41]

---

*   For a thorough and compelling description of this process, read Elisabeth Rosenthal's *An American Sickness*, pages 132–134.

Where there's a failed device, there's a recall. Where there's a recall, there's an injured or ill person, their family, and their medical bills. As an affected individual, or a loved one, there's very little you can do about it—this isn't Waffle House: you don't get medical care "on the house" if the equipment used on you is faulty.* You can sue, but good luck squeezing a dime from equipment manufacturers' highly paid and extremely aggressive legal teams. You can sign a petition and try to pursue legislation, but the equipment manufacturers are protected by several modest but competent lobbying organizations, including the Medical Device Manufacturers Association (MDMA).†

So lookalike device by lookalike device, pushy salesman by pushy salesman, device failure by device failure, costs pile up.

Pharmaceuticals

Then there's the pharmaceutical industry. It's easy to describe the ways the pharma industry jacks up costs thanks to the very public case of Martin Shkreli, the iconically smug pharma executive who bought up the rights to toxoplasmosis drug Daraprim‡ and increased its price per dose from $13.50 to $750 (about 56 times).[42] A light course of treatment—hypothetically, two pills a day for six weeks—would now

---

* Waffle House gets a lot of shit and none of it is deserved. I don't care if a fight breaks out. I can get hashbrowns scattered, smothered, diced, and capped at 4:15 AM on a Wednesday, and that's America to me. Everyone who works there deserves a union, a pension, and the same kind of respect we afford doctors and judges. Everyone else deserves this, too.

† I can't believe they got that initialism.

‡ A drug with no competitors that was, by all accounts, satisfactory at its job and first approved in 1953.

run somebody $63,000, up from $1,134.* One demographic for Daraprim is people with HIV/AIDS, who are fighting infection due to lowered immunoresponse—already a population that is extremely at risk.

Shkreli ultimately ended up in jail—but not because of this. The "Pharma Bro" only saw the inside of a courtroom because he defrauded *rich* people.† There's no law against jacking up drug prices for sick people. There's nothing legally wrong about making sure people who want their children to survive a rare disease pay until they bleed. In fact, it's encouraged! For all the uproar, all the media attention—the price of Daraprim, still owned by Shkreli's Turing Pharmaceuticals, *remains* $750.[43] Shkreli is notable only because he got in front of cameras: there are *hundreds*, if not *thousands*, of situations matched note for note.

Take, for example, the EpiPen. It's a little pen-shaped doodad that supplies epinephrine to people having an anaphylactic reaction, keeping them alive longer. It means life and death for a lot of people‡ and in 2004 it cost $53 to purchase. Ten years later, nothing about the pen had changed—except the price, which patent owner Mylan had sextupled to $300.[44] There was another typical round of media uproar, another round of how-dare-yous, Mylan posited that the price increases were necessary because of costs associated with new "branding," and nothing meaningful happened. Well—one meaningful thing happened. Mylan CEO Heather Bresch saw her salary rise 671 percent to $19 million.[45] And she used that money well: in the 2018 cycle, Mylan executives were among the largest contributors to West Virginia Democratic Senator Joe Manchin. The money stayed in the family: Bresch is Manchin's daughter.

---

* $1,134 is also too high.

†   AND because he threatened to reveal the Wu-Tang Secret. But mostly because he defrauded a hedge fund.

‡   Including me, a congenital "Indoors Kid"

One more everyday example of pharmaceutical price inflation is insulin. Insulin is an essential medicine for more than
7 million of the 20 million people with diabetes in the United
States. It's a miracle drug and a triumph of modern science—
even more so when you consider that when three Canadian
doctors invented it in 1923, they declined a million-dollar deal
from drugmaker Eli Lilly and instead sold its patent to the University of Toronto for one dollar apiece.*

Sadly, there's an unhappy ending to this story: immediately
after acquiring the patent, the University of Toronto licensed
it for free to several pharmaceutical manufacturers. This is understandable in light of the difficult start-up costs to synthesize
and replicate insulin in volume, especially at the time, but had
the unfortunate consequence of handing this drug to the very
corporations who are now helping to kill people with their
price increases. No good deed goes unpunished.

Since 2003, insulin has tripled in cost.[46] While there have
been developments in insulin quality and production technology, that cost increase applies even to insulin products
that haven't changed much. Some people are stuck paying
thousands of dollars a month for a medicine they used to be
able to afford. When people with diabetes can't afford their
insulin, they try to make it last longer—stretching two doses
into three, or going longer between doses.[47] Some people *do*
have insurance that covers insulin, but not the specific for-
mulation they need (or it imposes too high a co-pay to receive it). I've sat with people across America who need to use
Facebook groups to trade the insulin they can *afford* for they
insulin they *need*.

The price of a dose of Sanofi's Lantus, a brand of insulin,
rose 600 percent between 2001 and 2015. Curiously, it appears
to have increased by the same amounts, and at virtually the

---

* A Canadian dollar, at that—virtually free!

same rate, as Novo Nordisk's competing brand, Levemir.[48]

This past November, protestors in Boston gathered outside Sanofi, one of the "Big Three" insulin manufacturers in the United States. Two of them were women bearing urns. Within the urns were their children—the ashes of their children, who died while rationing insulin their families couldn't afford.[49]

Who killed these children? I wish there were a simple and direct answer; an accusation we could lay against a pair of feet; a body we could shake; a smirk we could wipe off a face. I wish our love and anger could be wielded like a weapon against a single enemy. Instead, there are many. Who are they?

Let us now name our foes one by one and draw out their web a strand at a time. We'll start with one triangular relationship you might not have realized has been lurking in the background every time you've filled a prescription.

A Brief Note on the Pretty Ugly Hate Machine of Pharmaceutical Costs

We've only scraped a fingernail's worth of gunk from the gaping, pestilent anus of the titanic pharmaceutical-industrial scam.* Here is a short detour into the dark world of *pharmacy benefit managers* (PBMs), one of the meanest, cruelest actors in American health finance.

There are three main bad guys whose various alliances and conflicts have created the unsustainable and inhumane shock of pharmaceutical costs, and even though two of them might gang up to point the finger at the third, *none* of them are up to any good.[†] Most of us know the first

---

* I'm trying very hard not to call everything a "[blank] industrial complex," but as you'll see, it's very difficult to resist.

† You might compare this dynamic to the Triple H vs. Chris Benoit vs. Shawn Michaels three-way feud, which culminated at Wrestlemania 20.

two: pharmaceutical companies and insurance companies. PBMs, the third, are less well-known.

PBMs are professional middlemen between insurance companies, pharmacies, and drug manufacturers. Insurers usually don't want to keep up with all the minutiae of the drugs available on the market: their trials, their alternatives, different courses of treatment available for a diagnosis, etc., so they contract a PBM to do this work for them. These contracts are signed in rooms with restricted electronic equipment so nobody can record or surveil what the contracts contain.*

At the core of this business relationship is this: if you have a diagnosis for which there is one cheap drug and one very expensive drug, your insurer would prefer that you choose the cheap drug. Think of the difference between name-brand and generic drugs. Name-brand Prozac can cost up to $500 for a set of 30 pills, while the generic fluoxetine might cost $17. Your insurer would prefer that you take fluoxetine. This is, frankly, a reasonable business position—but one which, when expanded, has severe, expensive, and harmful consequences for the people who need those drugs.

The PBM hires some pharmacists to assemble a list of preferred drugs and assigns them various tiers based on some measure of their "cost-effectiveness"—drugs that are cheaper to purchase, like generics, tend to go lower; drugs that are more expensive are put higher. The result is a list called a *formulary*, which is licensed to the insurer, along with adjustments to bring them in line

---

* There's a bill (the C-THRU Act) specifically addressing this: https://www.congress.gov/bill/115th-congress/senate-bill/637.

with coverage regulations in different states. This formulary is written into your insurance plan, and is why you are charged different co-pays for different tiers of medications—a drug on the bottom might be relatively inexpensive or free (some insurers offer "free generic drugs"), while a drug a tier up has a co-pay.

The PBM is also contracted to be the direct negotiator with pharmaceutical manufacturers. Since the PBM represents many insurers, it can bargain at scale to receive discounts from the manufacturers. A PBM can and will play rough, even removing a drug entirely from all its formularies if it doesn't think it's getting a sweet enough deal. (This is why your drugs might switch between coverage and non-coverage from year to year. It's this petty.) These deals come in two flavors: discounts and rebates. Discounts are what they sound like: directly lowered prices. Rebates are reimbursements from the manufacturer after purchase. These sound similar, but their functions are very different.

The rebate from the manufacturer might be paid to the PBM, the insurer, or the patient. Most commonly it's paid to the PBM, who keeps some and gives the rest to the insurer.[50] The insurer could give this remaining rebate to the patient to help pay the high costs of drugs, but they never do. (Worse, they usually set co-pays on the list price instead of the price after rebate, pushing unnecessary costs onto the patient.) On top of that, these rebates are recorded as general revenues instead of adjustments to drug spending—so when the insurer looks at its drug spending at the end of the year, the costs look much greater than the actual money spent. And so premiums go up.

Here are some ways this shakes out:

- PBMs will demand higher and higher rebates from manufacturers, who will then raise their list price to accommodate. This drives prices up.
- Sometimes, the PBM sets prices such that a patient pays *more* for a drug through their insurance co-pay than they would if they paid for it out of pocket with no insurance. This is called a "clawback." On top of that, until it was banned by Congress in October 2018, PBMs would enforce gag orders on pharmacists, forbidding them from *telling this to the patient.* It was estimated that, before the ban, almost a quarter of all drugs had these clawbacks.[51]
- Then there's the loathsome "spread," in which PBMs charge insurance companies a higher amount than what they reimburse the pharmacy or manufacturer, and keep the change. One study found that in Ohio, two PBMs billed Medicaid $200 million more than they paid pharmacies ($2.5 billion versus $2.3 billion.)[52] This went directly into their pockets.
- You might notice that rebates are the preferred transaction instead of direct discounts.[53] This has a few purposes, of which one is particularly foul. By offering rebates, including rebates directly to customers, manufacturers keep list prices high. That is, Dongerman's Drugs might sell a pill for $800, but offer the insurer a rebate of $700. The insurance company only pays a net amount of $100, but the list price stays at $800. Since insurance

co-pays are often set on list price instead of the after-rebate price, this means you pay out the nose for expensive drugs you need.* Your insurance company might win a substantial rebate for that drug—but none of it is passed to you.

- State Medicaid programs pay a discount on the lowest prices at which a manufacturer sells a drug to PBMs and insurers. Until very recently, the prices Medicaid used were based on list price, not net price. Since Medicaid is funded by both the state and the federal government, it has a much more limited pool of resources to draw from, and sky-high drug prices can put an entire state program at stake. This recently led to a fiasco in Washington over groundbreaking hepatitis C medication Sovaldi, a course of which Medicaid had to purchase for $80,000.[54] (Government healthcare agencies that can negotiate drug prices get this drug for $18,000 a course, and in India a course of Sovaldi costs $336.)[55]

- At the same time, the state of Washington is, like virtually every other state, battling a rash of opioid-use disorder; hepatitis C, which can be transmitted through shared needle use, is a comorbidity of opioid-use disorder. (Comorbidities are simultaneously occurring diseases or disorders that interact to make the treatment of the other more difficult or complicated.) The austerity politics of Medicaid

---

* Or, more frequently, you are *not* able to afford paying out the nose for an expensive drug you need.

collided with the outbreak of hepatitis C and its sky-high cost of treatment, and ultimately the Washington Medicaid program began restricting access to hepatitis treatment unless a patient was already deathly ill. Thousands were condemned to grow sick and suffer. (Washington was later sued for this practice and was forced to expand its coverage to all Medicaid recipients, at significant cost to the state and its tax coffers.)[56]

PBMs and insurers have begun acquiring each other: CVS and Aetna merged in 2018; Optum and UnitedHealth did the same. The PR flacks for these corporations announce the amazing savings that the vertical integration of these corporations will produce. Cool! Will any of these savings be passed on to the patient? Absolutely not. The whole output of this big awful machine, this jousting between PBMs and insurers and drug manufacturers, is virtually a mass corporate conspiracy to soak Medicare, Medicaid, and you.

Nobody here is a "good guy," and everyone uses patients to their advantage. Sometimes manufacturers will fund patient advocacy groups (ex., "Mothers Against Cat Head Disease") to lobby Congress to relax FDA regulation on drug manufacturers (so the patient advocacy groups can get the drugs they need for Cat Head Disease sooner).[57] Sometimes insurers will help fund patient advocacy groups to protest drug manufacturers, blaming them for the skyrocketing cost of the drugs they produce. It's a mucky, murky water—and however you sift it, it surfaces something awful for patients. No patient is ever wrong for protesting, but this interplay between patient interest and corporate interest all leads to rising costs for drugs, both out of the manufacturer and out of your wallet, year after year.

PBMs don't get much time in the spotlight, and they like it that way. But alongside the actors I've already laid out and the ones I'll lay out next, they're as bad as anyone—an absolute Frankenstein of the excesses and unnecessary paperwork of American health finance, rampaging through the villages of our prescription prices.

Hospitals

Last in our survey of cost increasers are *hospitals*. Amid a national wave of closures of Medicaid clinics and local community clinics, hospitals increasingly serve as the first (or only) point of entry for sick people to access medical care in America. They obviously provide an essential service to their patients and often serve as hubs for healthcare programs in their communities. By and large, the doctors, nurses, social workers, and every other on-the-ground staff member of these hospitals are not causing problems for American healthcare. The same cannot be said for the institutions they work for—which often do not reflect the saints after which many of them name themselves.

And not all hospitals are the same. Some are hardscrabble rural operations in conservative states that treat at their own expense uninsured patients put into the "Medicaid gap" (Do you live in a state that refused to expand Medicaid? Are you too poor to qualify for the ACA but ineligible for your state's austere Medicaid program? You have been left to rot in the Medicaid gap). Other hospitals are the $8 billion Cleveland

Clinic—one of the nation's preeminent "prestige" hospitals, with lavish luxury suites and concierge services for its billionaire and royalty clientele (a "palace away from home"),[58] built in the middle of, and walled off from, a desperately segregated, impoverished, and *sick* neighborhood.[59] The people of the neighborhood surrounding a world-class Cleveland Clinic have a life expectancy seven years shorter than the people of wealthier neighborhoods literally a few minutes to the east.[60]

Some hospitals are like the University of Pittsburgh Medical Center (UPMC) in Pittsburgh, Pennsylvania. On top of being a nationally renowned facility, UPMC is the largest healthcare provider, largest employer, and a major insurer in Pittsburgh. Unsurprisingly, giving a corporation total dominion over a community hasn't resulted in good health outcomes or a just healthcare landscape. UPMC pulls in almost $16 billion a year in revenue—and even after spending billions of dollars, maintains almost $400 million in operating profit.* This profit is driven by its insurance product and its aggressive expansion across the county; UPMC builds (or acquires) facilities and reopens them as part of the UPMC hospital complex, which means these facilities now charge expensive hospital rates for providing almost the same services—sometimes even by the same people—as they used to. Despite it all, UPMC is a not-for-profit corporation, and it wields its status to avoid paying taxes—going so far as claiming it has *no direct employees* in order to get out of employment tax.[61] UPMC even avoids paying its water bills, because the state can't shut down the utilities of a hospital.[62]

So what does a huge multibillion-dollar health complex like UPMC do with all this money? It opens food pantries for the employees who can't afford to eat on UPMC wages.[63]

---

* An operating Earnings Before Interest, Depreciation and Amortization (EBIDA) of $483 million in 2018.

With this context, it may not surprise you to learn that hospitals are in many ways the primary drivers of healthcare costs in the United States.[64] In the American hospital, a given inpatient procedure—that is, a procedure for which the patient is admitted to the hospital—costs 40 percent more than the exact same procedure performed on the same type of patient when performed in France.[65] In California, one study found that the cost of an appendectomy—a relatively simple procedure with few points of complication—can range from $1,500 to $182,000, without necessarily corresponding to a difference in patient health or difficulty.[66] There's no good reason for this kind of massive variation from hospital to hospital. It just happens because hospitals *can* do it, it's been happening for at least 30 years,[*] and nobody's gonna stop 'em.[†]

But even if you don't live in Cleveland or Pittsburgh, the size and weight of these hospital chains affect you in personal ways. Intimate ways. Let's consider the relationship, and the contrast, between primary care and hospitals.

Primary care is the kind of familiar, personal healthcare you get from your family physician or general practitioner (or primary care provider). In many cases, PCPs help people navigate the broader or more comprehensive healthcare system—

---

[*]   There's a famous study in Vermont (a relatively homogenous state) that found massive discrepancies in tonsillectomies from county to county, even when there was no substantial difference between the populations examined. Some people just like performing tonsillectomies more than others, and some hospitals encourage physicians to perform surgeries more enthusiastically than others do.

   There's another famous study in which a sample group of children with sore throats were brought to a set doctors in NYC, and half were prescribed tonsillectomies. Those who weren't prescribed tonsillectomies were brought back to another doctor in the set, and again, about half were prescribed tonsillectomies. Those who remained were once again returned to the doctors—and, once again, about half were prescribed tonsillectomies.

   These anecdotes demonstrate the ability of providers to influence medical spending not only by setting costs but by creating demand as well.

[†]   Yet.

like when you go to your family doctor to figure out whether your earache warrants visiting an oncologist (cancer doctor) or an ENT (ear, nose, and throat doctor). At its best, primary care is composed of physicians in their communities—people who intimately understand the health needs of the people around them. It's high-volume, it's low-margin, and even though it's essential, generally it's not super-profitable.

In a country where healthcare is treated like a commodity,* this essential care isn't profitable. This has grave consequences. It's bad for doctors, it's bad for patients, and ultimately, it drives healthcare costs up across the whole country.

There're a lot of things happening here, so for the purposes of explaining it, let's think of it as a three-step process. First, PCPs get squeezed by the market forces surrounding primary care and either retire or seek acquisition. Next, hospitals buy up clinics that provide primary care and become patients' first contact points for their healthcare needs—now at hospital-level prices. Last, the resulting financial and geographic barriers cause people to postpone seeking the healthcare they need, or they don't get it at all.

Let's break these down one at a time.

First: PCPs get squeezed by the market.

This is a systemic problem in American health finance: we don't pay primary care providers enough, so when they eventually retire or otherwise close up shop, there's nobody available to replace them. (Even though PCPs might make much more than you or I make,† they—alongside psychiatrists and pediatricians—exit medical school with a few hundred thousand dollars in debt and make almost three times less than other kinds of specialist doctors like orthopedic surgeons.)[67]

---

* Though it shouldn't!

† If you make more money than the average doctor, please purchase a second copy of this book. Thank you.

This is driven by two things: the shortcomings of health-care billing models that undervalue the "compassionate labor" behind primary care, and the efforts of lobbying groups to push money away from primary care toward specialty care.

What makes for a good primary care provider? It's not just technical precision. In a lot of cases, being a good PCP requires emotional connection, trust, and more than a little bit of social work with patients. The trouble is, each of these takes time, and time doesn't get you paid. Most PCPs are paid on a fee-for-service plan, in which doctors make a list of all the material things they provide a patient ("office visit," "flu shot," "lanced cyst," etc.), sum up the resulting costs, and fax it to the patient's insurance company. This sounds sensible, but the model presumes that an "office visit" is the same from person to person. A patient who can be in and out of your office in 20 minutes with a simple question and quick prescription gets you paid the same as someone who needs 15 minutes to get up on the bed and who has a lot of questions and concerns about how to manage her and her children's health—even if her visit takes three times as long. (And this, of course, presumes they both have an insurance plan.) If you're working in a poorer, more rural, or sicker area, you're more likely to have patients who need more time and slow compassion. Because insurers don't pay very much for office visits,[68] PCPs face a lot of pressure to move through as many patients as they can, as quickly as they can.

This is exacerbated by how little time doctors have to work with patients. Nationwide, half the average doctor's time is spent dealing with billing systems, insurer paperwork, and electronic health records.[69] Only one of these—health records—are of any actual usefulness to a patient's health.

Then there's the shifting of payment away from primary care providers to specialty providers. This is driven by some nerd-club parliamentary procedure shit. In short: every year, the American Medical Association advises Medicare's RVS Update Committee (RUC) about the relative difficulty and cost of different medical procedures. This advice is used to determine how much to pay for each procedure—and since virtually every insurer in the United States bases its payment levels on Medicare's, the RUC ultimately determines payment levels for every provider in America. The AMA's advisory team is nominally a representative body for every kind of doctor in the United States: PCPs have a representative, hand surgeons have a representative, cardiologists have a representative, and so on. That sounds good, except that PCPs compose approximately half of America's doctors.[70] If you're familiar with America's electoral college, you might know where this is going. Uh-oh!

It turns out that since every specialist has a representative on this body, they prefer to give advice that benefits specialists as a class over PCPs and everyone else. Take knee replacements, for example. The AMA committee might determine that there are two kinds of knee replacements: an "easy" kind, which happens half the time and should cost half as much as the previous standard for knee surgery, and a "hard" kind, which describes the other half of cases and should be paid twice as much. On the surface, Medicare likes this proposal: since the AMA committee claims both surgeries happen half the time, Medicare's net spending should stay the same. Right? So it accepts the recommendations from the expert body and writes it into Medicare's payment list ("fee schedule").

Except—as soon as this payment scheme is enforced, every hospital in America, every billing department in the country, begins billing every knee surgery at the more expensive classification as often as possible. Medicare pays more, insurers pay more, primary care providers don't get their share of the pie, and medical costs rise.*

All of this compounds upon itself. America is facing a short-

---

* This is an insanely compressed hypothetical that describes a real, but much longer, more complicated, and more *infuriating* process. For a book about this entire process and the many, many more that comprise the RUC's activity, read Miriam J. Laugesen's brilliant *Fixing Medical Prices*.

age of primary care providers as PCPs age out and nobody can afford to replace them. The United States has the J-1 visa for doctors from other countries (usually countries where it is much cheaper to become a doctor), but that's a Band-Aid solution that deprives other countries of their own medical workforce.

This PCP shortage is an entirely man-made problem. In fact, in the eighties and early nineties, America feared it would soon have *too many* doctors![71] The *New Yorker* even ran cartoons about doctors waiting in breadlines. Clinton-era medical policy tightened funding for residency programs with an eye on "intelligently" narrowing the number of doctors in the United States and shifting patients to more "efficient" HMOs, those narrow and restrictive insurer provider networks you've probably found yourself confused or frustrated by at least once in your insured life.

As a result we now have an extremely expensive medical training program that actively promotes specialty care as being a superior aspiration and denigrates primary care as the domain of the less intellectual or ambitious. This tension exacerbates health inequities in rural or poor areas, keeps doctors from pursuing medicine that isn't specialty care in places that aren't urban areas, leads to massive doctor shortages in areas where doctors are needed most, and drives up medical prices.*

Second: Hospitals buy up clinics that provide primary care and become patients' first contact points for their healthcare needs—now at hospital-level prices.

Hospitals get paid an average of $2,000 a night for an inpa-

---

* If you watch daytime TV, you might have heard of something called "direct primary care," in which a PCP contracts directly with a patient for a set monthly fee. It can be useful in very specific scenarios, but does not scale to resolve any of the structural problems primary care is facing. It's good for the provider and can be fine for the patient, but only if the patient can afford it as a *supplement* to insurance—often, it's marketed as a replacement for insurance altogether, which is utterly inadequate. It also only works in areas where PCPs are relatively abundant—direct primary care has nothing for rural, poor, or areas with PCP shortages. In short, it's a Band-Aid solution for people who can already afford insurance.

tient stay.* This is the proverbial "good stuff," and it means that the hospital corporation's job is, in many respects, to get as many inpatient admissions as possible. There's a little truism in health finance known as Roemer's Law, which posits that any hospital bed that is built will be filled, regardless of need in the surrounding community. In fact, there's evidence that a given doctor who works at two hospitals will adjust the rate at which they admit people to inpatient care depending on which hospital they're currently working at, and how aggressively it encourages its doctors to admit.[72]

To the hospital executive, the legions of primary care clinics around them represent an incredible business opportunity. Some of the patients who go to these clinics are ultimately admitted to a hospital or a surgery center. Unless this is a one-hospital town, some percentage of those patients is being admitted to a *different* hospital from the one headed by the executive. What a waste of money! Why should the hospital executive waste her time letting doctors provide cheap primary care outside her hospital when they could be pushing those patients directly into her hospital? So the hospital moves in—merging with smaller hospitals, buying clinics outright, and sometimes shutting them down afterward. It's big business: 90 hospital merger deals were announced in 2018, with a total deal size of $36.8 billion.[73†]

To the low-paid primary care provider, this represents a chance to ease out of being self-employed and make a higher income with more consistency (and outsource some of the paperwork to the hospital's massive billing department). To the hospital, this represents a chance to ensure that any patient who needs inpatient care (or any patient whose insurer could be convinced they need inpatient care) is admitted to the owner hospital and its billing department. This is also an op-

---

* Dividing average charge per inpatient visit by average length of inpatient stay

† I'm defining deal size as the sum of seller valuations. (Sellers are the smaller of two entities in a merger.)

portunity to leverage the hospital's size and negotiating power
with insurers to use the existing clinic to charge hospital-level
prices for the exact same services it used to provide—an average cost increase of 14 percent, simply for being under hospital
ownership.[74]

(This presumes that the patients in question have insurance. Hospital executives aren't interested in getting the business of poor or uninsured people. Unsurprisingly, the hospital
merger business has failed to improve the conditions of rural
clinics and rural hospitals closing across the country. And in
the event that a hospital's acquisition *does* bring in more uninsured patients, privately owned hospitals exercise the privilege
of being able to turn away unprofitable patients in non-emergency situations.)

Third, and last: People get the healthcare they need later, or
they don't get it at all. Now that low-paid primary care clinics have closed their doors, or been snatched up by corporate
hospitals, a few things happen. Patients who need healthcare
find that their options are limited. Rural patients have seen the
process of clinic consolidation and closure play out for about
two decades, now exacerbated by hospital closures (especially
in states that chose not to expand Medicaid as part of the ACA).
No providers are moving in to replace them, and it's not uncommon to find large swaths of the country where a person needs to
travel over an hour to get to the nearest hospital. In urban areas,
having to go to the hospital instead of a local clinic (or having
a local clinic that's booked solid because there's nowhere else
to go) means patients face a massive bill every time they need
healthcare—exponentially more so if they're not insured. This
keeps patients from seeking healthcare at all when they need it.

The irony of primary care being relatively inexpensive and
therefore difficult to sustain is that it's essential in preventing serious healthcare complications—and serious healthcare
costs—down the road. Catching an illness or disease early is

both much better for a patient's quality of life and also, by preventing the need for catastrophic emergency care from an untreated condition, much better for their pocketbook.

Because no matter how difficult you make it to access healthcare, at some urgent, traumatic, and dire point, the need for healthcare can overcome financial and geographic barriers, no matter how disastrous the outcome for the patient. That's when the real cost sinks in. People who might have been able to get on a diabetes treatment plan if they'd been screened early in their disease instead wait until their feet swell to the size of chickens before seeking care. People with strange lumps and pains don't learn they have cancer until they're well into stage II or stage III. Wounds are "walked off" until they fester and turn severely infected. In all of these situations, the cost of care is *multiples* higher for later care.*

One anecdote traces this whole cycle. Johns Hopkins is one of the best hospitals in the world (along with Cleveland Clinic, mentioned earlier, and Mayo Clinic in Rochester, Minnesota). It has a dominant position in Baltimore as both a massive healthcare provider and an employer. Slowly, in its shadow, primary care clinics and community health centers have been acquired, closed, or shut down, particularly in poor neighborhoods. But the residents of those poor neighborhoods still need healthcare—now Johns Hopkins's emergency department has a constant stream of traffic—including a large number of people with non-emergency problems who just have nowhere else to go.

Pretend you're the Johns Hopkins CEO. How would you handle this problem? Would you build an urgent care center? Would you open local clinics in the neighborhoods of the people who are filling your hospital with non-emergencies? That's what I might do.

---

* This is not to say that "universal preventive care" is a solution. It isn't. A lot of people who can't afford to get screened for diabetes can't afford the medications that are required if the test comes out positive.

And that's why I'm not the CEO of Johns Hopkins! Instead, the hospital built an urgent-care clinic inside the ED—and charges ED prices for its use. For many patients, there is still nowhere else to turn.

★ ★ ★

With these examples, I've shone not a torch but a very small penlight across the incomprehensible hulking mass of these industries. Some of these grifts are massive and structural; some are tiny, personal, small enough to fit in your palm or under your tongue. The scams of American healthcare are all very tightly interwoven; they are like a hundred thousand bloated rats, some the size of an infant's fist, others the size of the night sky, each one eating another's tail: an impenetrable, writhing, nauseating mass. This is an ecosystem upon which you and I and everyone we love are utterly dependent for our survival. It's one that avails itself of any opportunity to squeeze us for just a little more profit. With such a dependent customer base, and a government that has at virtually every juncture chosen to enable those who wish us harm, is it any wonder costs are out of control?

Of course not.

There are two wretched and fundamental truths to American healthcare:

- If you are a payer, like an insurance company, *it is not profitable* to insure people who are sick; and
- If you are a provider, like a hospital, or a pharma company, it is *extremely profitable* to charge sick people as much as possible, as late as possible, so long as somebody is footing the bill.

We have built upon these jagged rocks the loathsome church of American healthcare, in which the question of "Who gets to receive healthcare, and when?"—or, rather, "Whose suffering matters?"—is determined by private profitability.

This whole situation scares the bejesus out of everyone involved, particularly the insurers. Insurers are interested in finding ways to avoid these rising costs. Sometimes that means refusing to pay for claims outright—it's certainly happened to you or someone you love. (It has happened to me *over* and *over* and *over* again. When it happens to you, know that your first step should always be to *appeal to the insurer*. If that doesn't work, you can *appeal to your state's insurance commission*.) Before the Affordable Care Act, this dynamic meant that private insurers on the individual market would just refuse to cover people who were or who were likely to get sick or be expensive—you know the phrase "preexisting conditions."

None of this was enough to bring costs down. So the insurance industry and their hired academics* formed a new monster from the muck, and in the 1970s introduced America to the idea of "consumer-driven" healthcare.

"SKIN IN THE GAME": PUNISHING PEOPLE FOR GETTING SICK

Consumer-driven healthcare describes the idea that you should make *consumers†* pay more for the costs of their own healthcare; that the patient needs to have more of their own

---

* Many health policy academics are wonderful people who work hard to better the lives of the people around them through their research. But not all. No matter how heinous the policy, no matter how urgent the consequences, there will always be a health policy academic who is ready to submit a paper about it for grant money. Their job is only to measure the size of the hole in the levee, even as the oncoming water threatens to drown us all.

† "Consumers" is libertarian for "people." A loathsome term when talking about healthcare.

"skin in the game" so they make efficient consumer purchasing choices. This ideology is fundamental to the problems in American healthcare and the pain you've felt in your own life—if you want a single "bad guy" for the book, here it is—so I'd like to discuss it at length.

Doesn't the patient literally have their skin in the game to begin with? you may wonder. Yes, absolutely. We all make healthcare purchasing choices with our literal, visceral well-being (or that of our family) in mind. However, this kind of decision-making is not profitable to insurance companies, so they've tried to force us into changing it.

At the core of this "consumer-driven" movement is a study conducted between 1974–1982 that examined what happened when people were made to pay for their own healthcare—up to this point, co-pays weren't common. Some test subjects kept their insurance plans with no co-pay, some were given small co-pays, and some were given large ones. It turns out, this study found, that when people have to pay healthcare costs they can't afford, they seek out less healthcare.[75] This is bad for the patients, this is bad for the families, but it's pretty good for the insurers because it means they have to pay out fewer claims.

Each actor recognizes the shock and horror of rising healthcare costs but insists they can't be the first to do anything about it (otherwise they'd lose profit). They then aggressively spend money to make sure our legislators feel similarly. Yet costs continue to increase. So with all other options exhausted, the only party left who can be manipulated is the "consumer"—so the costs are pushed to them. To you. To us. When there is nowhere else to profit, our bodies are set on fire.

This cruel ideology introduces the idea of "wrongness" to healthcare—wrongness defined not by its relationship to the patient, but whether it's bad for the insurer and the insurer's profit sheets. The insurer becomes the ultimate moral arbiter, a dickweed God, that determines that there are *wrong* doctors, *wrong* clinics, and *wrong* hospitals, wrong because they either wouldn't give the insurance company a good enough deal or because they have a habit of billing more than the insurer is willing to pay for a frequent procedure. If there are too many *wrong* doctors in a community, the insurer imposes correction by refusing to pay for any healthcare they provide. This creates a big scattered maze of doctors: there are some doctors whom you can visit and have your care covered; others, you must either avoid or pay calamitous fees. Patients must then map out the constellation of "right" providers and seek healthcare at their own peril. In this manner, the insurer's financial concerns impose a fucked-up moral framework upon the patient's choices. A patient who chooses to see the *wrong* doctors is making a *wrong* choice, and therefore must be punished with increased or overwhelming costs, so as to encourage them to make the "right" choice next time. Perhaps the example of those who chose *wrongly* will serve as a warning—like a bleached skull speared atop a post outside an orc camp.

Certainly providers *do* overcharge; hospitals *do* seek to squeeze as much as they can out of the insurance company. Thus the insurers, who need profit like patients need air and water, have a legitimate and reasonable point. But that their point can only be expressed at the expense of the patient is proof of the moral illegitimacy of the whole industry.

This is the idea behind the "insurance network" concept, which determines which doctors you can see and which you can't—and its innovative new-generation offshoot, the "narrow network," which is just like a regular network except smaller and worse. Innovation!

This is why your deductibles and co-pays increase every year. Because once you are made to suffer for making a "wrong" choice, once you are liable for healthcare costs set so astronomically out of your reach, you will (the "consumer-driven healthcare" movement promises) be transformed into a "smart shopper," somehow, and through the power of the free market or whatever, you will shop around and not get "unnecessary"* or "too expensive" care; you will find the cheapest emergency department if you get hit by a car; you will, like, Yelp your surgeons; and all of this will, somehow, drive prices down.

That's absurd. We have internalized the language that just protects insurer profits. Because insurance companies claim they can't afford the rising costs of healthcare, their brilliant solution is to force more and more of those costs onto *us*. This is why 28 percent of people with employer-sponsored insurance plans spend $6,000 a year on premiums for insurance plans with deductibles over $2,200—or *$19,000 in premiums* with a $4,500 deductible if you have a family[76]—while 40 percent of Americans can't afford a $400 medical emergency.[77]

You know what's even worse than that? *It doesn't even work!* No, when we are forced to pay for healthcare costs we can't afford, we don't become better shoppers. Instead, we don't seek out any healthcare whatsoever. We don't do this "rationally," by declining only the most expensive care—no, we just don't get primary care. We don't seek preventive care. We ignore that rash, we try not to look at that tumor, we think away that chest pain. Because insurance companies demand we bear the burden of increasing healthcare costs, we are forced to lose our bodies slowly and then all at once. We are made to watch passively as our bodies twist into time bombs—to spend our lives pruning the ever-branching anxiety of recognizing the illnesses we know we can do nothing about—until they explode; until we have a heart attack and leave our kids behind.

And yet, despite their protestations about the indignities of the healthcare market, insurance companies are raking in unimaginable profits—higher now than ever in recent mem-

---

* Implicit in all this is the idea that there's a whole world of people out there who are getting, like, recreational knee replacements.

ory. Copays, deductibles, networks, all the bilge and detritus of the "consumer-driven" movement—this is their attempt to scare us into delaying our own expensive care until they're no longer responsible for the bills. It's a calculated maneuver to extract as much as possible from everyone and give as little as they can in return. Consumer-driven healthcare is, at this point, just the rules of the game, and until we wipe out the whole game altogether, we have to square up with it.

This sucks.

Before we talk about what must be done, I'd like to talk about what *has* been tried—and why it didn't work.

THE AFFORDABLE CARE ACT

So what do you do? How do you square the rampant increase of healthcare costs with the fact that insuring sick people isn't profitable?

Well, if you're the Democrats, you collaborate with the conservative Heritage Foundation think tank[78] to offer us the **Affordable Care Act (ACA)**, which is, fundamentally, the massive subsidization of the private insurance industry with public money. The ACA is a big bargain, a plaintive wail: *Please, please*, it asks, *how many billions of dollars do we need to give you so you stop kicking sick people off their insurance plans?*

The ACA was a massive bill that included hundreds of new regulations, adjustments, carrots, and sticks for healthcare providers, insurance companies, and everyone in between. It derives from a (myopic) school of policy in which legislative goals are determined as a function of some statistic: "too many children are hungry," for example, or "too many teens are in ska bands." In this case, the core problem of the ACA was: too many people are uninsured.

This is an objectively correct assessment, as even a single person being uninsured is one person too many. And so, it was far beyond "too many" people who were uninsured. Throughout the 1990s and into the 2000s, about 16 percent of the non-elderly (and thus non-Medicare) population was uninsured.[79] That's about 50 million people.[80] This is a *cataclysmic* number of uninsured people. Many of these uninsured people had jobs, or worked *multiple* jobs, and were refused insurance through their employer(s). Many lived in states where Medicaid eligibility was so restrictive that they were categorically denied coverage. Others had diabetes or had had cancer in the past or had a mental illness for which insurance companies refused to sell them insurance plans—or would only do so at impossibly high premiums.

There were two main prongs in the ACA's approach to resolve these problems: *Medicaid expansion* and the regulation, development, and subsidization of the *individual insurance marketplace*. Between these two efforts, the ACA drove down the uninsured population in America from almost 18 percent to 10 percent.[81]

Medicaid expansion was responsible for the bulk of the newly insured,* with individual insurance picking up the rest.[82] If expanding Medicaid worked so well, why did some states with lots of uninsured people choose not to do it? This wasn't an intended outcome of the ACA. We discussed before that Medicaid is funded jointly by the state and federal government and that this meant states could set their own eligibility criteria for Medicaid. Medicaid expansion under the ACA was intended to set nationwide standards for Medicaid eligi-

---

* Actual numbers are a little tricky to define, because it requires answering questions like, "If a child who was eligible for Medicaid was enrolled because their parent was also made eligible under the ACA, does this count as a normal Medicaid enrollment or an ACA enrollment?" Either way, Medicaid is accountable for a maximum of 75 percent of the drop in uninsurance since the ACA went into effect, and I'm inclined to put it closer to there than 50 percent.

bility, instead of leaving that determination up exclusively to the states, which tended to be more restrictive—especially in poorer and more conservative areas. Under the original intent of the ACA, the federal government would fund the difference in spending between pre-ACA Medicaid programs and an expanded Medicaid program that accepted anyone with an income up to 138 percent of the federal poverty line (about $17,000 if you're a single person).*

Conservative states, in a show of ideological contempt for poor and disabled people and people of color, sued. Then came the Supreme Court. *NFIB v. Sebelius* determined that Congress had the power to enact most parts of the ACA, but that it was incapable of mandating that state Medicaid programs had to adopt the new eligibility guidelines. That's why several states have refused to do so, and why Medicaid eligibility criteria still varies from state to state. It is a barbaric decision and it permits states to refuse desperately needed federal money, to actively harm their people, for reasons of political tribalism.

In the intervening years, several states have chosen to expand Medicaid. This is a mitzvah. Some have done this through their elected officials—fine. Others have done this with restrictions like work requirements—shameful. Yet others have done so not through their elected officials but through state referendums, mass mobilizations of the population. This is nothing short of amazing. We'll discuss one such state, Idaho, at the end of this book.

Then there's the individual insurance marketplace. It's how over 20 million people have become insured since the ACA—including me, and many of my friends, who stack multiple part-time jobs on top of each other but receive benefits from none of them.[83] It works like this, generally: the federal government

---

* The portion of the funding covered by the federal government would decrease over time, presumably as states got accustomed to the cost and reaped the (significant) economic benefits of lower uninsurance.

mandates that all people must have insurance.* If you don't have public insurance, that means you gotta buy private insurance—and you might turn to the ACA marketplace to do so.

Every year, insurers who want to compete in the ACA marketplace submit the insurance plans they'd like to sell. Regardless of whether they use the ACA's marketplace infrastructure, they need to cover a list of essential health benefits (EHBs)—basically a "bare minimum" guideline for what an insurance plan might cover. This EHB policy is unequivocally good. Before the ACA, insurers would sell "junk plans"—very cheap insurance plans that capped payouts at a couple thousand dollars or that didn't cover broad swaths of treatment—meaning that people walked around *thinking* they were insured (and at a bargain price!) but found themselves tens or even hundreds of thousands of dollars in debt when something serious happened. EHBs mean that no matter *how* crummy your plan is otherwise, it at least covers hospitalizations, maternal care, and (ostensibly, but not in practice) mental health services.

Once the plans are in, with their projected prices, the ACA calculates a percentage of your income it thinks is reasonable for you to pay for insurance.† It then offers subsidies to you based upon two things: the price of the second-cheapest silver-tier plan (plans are tiered based on how much cost they push on you) offered by insurers in your area,‡ and your declared expected income.

---

* This was one of the core ideas challenged in the *NFIB v. Sebelius* lawsuit. The Court found that the federal government could, in fact, mandate the purchase of insurance. Over time, this mandate has not been enforced, making it barely a mandate.

† These subsidies were determined on the premise that the American family should spend 10 percent of its income on insurance costs. This is ludicrous—a family making $70,000 a year doesn't have $7,000 to spend on insurance premiums, especially when 40 percent of Americans can't afford a $400 emergency!

‡ This is potentially an area of *mass* corporate collusion.

Subsidies are available to people who make between 138 percent and 400 percent of the federal poverty level ($12,140 in 2018), which translates to a range of $16,574–$48,560. If you make less than $16,574, the ACA presumes you are on Medicaid.

If you're on the low end of that range, almost all of your insurance plan purchase might be subsidized—your co-pays might be subsidized too. If you're on the upper end, subsidies can get pretty flimsy. A $12 subsidy doesn't feel great when your insurance plan costs $500 a month.

But if you make just one dollar over $48,560, you don't get bupkis. You have to pay for that whole insurance premium on your own. And after you get the insurance, better not need to go to the doctor *too* frequently—because the co-pays are also all on you.

If this doesn't make sense, once again, don't worry. It doesn't. It's a plan designed by nerds who like looking at spreadsheets so much that they figured everyone else would enjoy it as well,* and that it might be a good way to determine who is permitted to live and die in America. It isn't a plan designed by *anyone* who has ever gone hungry to feed their kids or anyone who lives in Section 8 housing or anyone who has ever been to prison.

And those marketplace subsidies? They go directly to the insurance companies.

*   *   *

I should withdraw my fangs from the ACA for a moment. It's important to identify where it *succeeded*. Because the ACA *did* succeed. It's just that the ACA's vision of a just world was one in which the government's job is to help private companies profit from insuring the uninsured *instead* of creating a world

---

* Ooh, shopping on the ACA marketplace and calculating my subsidy, one can imagine them giggling. What a thrill!

in which its people don't need to be uninsured in the first place—an inequity that the government *could* work to resolve reasonably simply. The ACA would prefer to rein in the excesses and abuses of the healthcare industries by guaranteeing their *profitability* and asking for small favors instead of listening to the screaming of the American people and acting. It is utterly convinced that the *problems* are bad, but that the *causes* of those problems are good and need billions of dollars in public bailout money.[84] The ACA is like a health policy conference asking "How Do We Cost-Effectively Improve Mental Health Outcomes for Children in Prison?" instead of asking why we put children in prison in the first place.

But I was talking about successes. First and foremost: The ACA's greatest success was the expansion of Medicaid. Despite legal roadblocks thrown in its way, expansion was by far the simplest part of the ACA and, if decreasing the uninsured rate is the goal, the most successful. In states that chose to expand Medicaid,* we saw a *6.1 percent* reduction in the mortality rate. That's *11.1 percent* among communities of color.[85] The reasons why are understood: these people have been systematically, if not violently, denied access to care in the first place. Even the relatively meager expansion of Medicaid helps people seek essential care when they need it.

Another accomplishment of the ACA was cementing the idea of "preexisting conditions" in the American vocabulary—as well as the idea that denying someone insurance *because* of them is immoral. For decades, people who had lost their jobs because of illness were unable to enroll in new insurance plans specifically *because* of that illness. And virtually nobody spoke

---

*   To date, 37 states (including D.C.) have chosen to expand Medicaid. Fourteen states have yet to expand Medicaid: Wyoming, South Dakota, Kansas, Wisconsin, Missouri, Oklahoma, Texas, Mississippi, Tennessee, Alabama, Georgia, South Carolina, North Carolina, and Florida: https://www.kff.org/medicaid/issue-brief/status-of-state-medicaid-expansion-decisions-interactive-map/.

about it—well, at least, nobody who got to be on TV. (Perhaps mainstream media coverage of structural problems that directly affect health and well-being is lacking.) These days—especially after the ACA repeal attempts of 2017—protections for people with preexisting conditions have to be at least nominally respected, even by the Republicans who seek to gut them.*

That's a hell of a difference from American health politics before 2008. But it's not enough. Costs keep increasing, quality of care stagnates—or worsens—for the most vulnerable people among us, and 31 million people remain uninsured. People are still dying from eminently preventable conditions because they're too poor—or the wrong *kind* of poor—to afford their healthcare costs.

Now—it is accurate to argue that the work of the ACA was hindered by the Republican Party during Obama's presidency and is being actively suffocated by Trump's administration. But it is inaccurate to imply that the ACA "would have worked" on its own, if not for the interference of other parties. The ACA was at best a life preserver for a healthcare system that is desperately failing its patients and that condemns the poor, the sick, and the disabled. It subsidized private companies enough to let poor people have insurance, but it didn't do anything to make that insurance *good*, or less difficult for people to use.† Even if it were larger, or if it were to have proceeded unfettered, it simply did not do very much to change

---

* There's a certain irony to the fact that these really took center stage only after the Republicans tried to gut the bill under Trump. I like to joke that Paul Ryan was the first person to actually try to sell the Affordable Care Act to the American public, but the Republicans certainly prompted the response from Americans that preexisting conditions were a nonnegotiable part of the ACA.

† That's why you observe the very real and heartbreakingly widespread phenomenon, even under the ACA, of poor people or people with disabilities having to divorce their partners or sell their houses or other assets so they can use Medicaid, which gives them the care they need without the grinding cost-sharing which would make private insurance plans unusuable.

the trajectory of the broader system. We have been given a series of complicated Band-Aids we barely understand, but our deep and gangrenous wounds have not been treated.

America has privileged corporate profit over the health of its people. You, me, and virtually everyone we know cannot afford the costs of staying alive. When confronted with this tension, America seeks to *rationalize* it—by forking more money over to companies—instead of improve it. The ACA failed in the pursuit of *health justice*. Perhaps it never set its gaze there at all.

THE MOST DANGEROUS PLACE

There are grave consequences for this failure.

Today, among so-called "developed countries," America is *the most dangerous place* to be sick.[86]*

Among peer countries, America is the most dangerous place to be Black. Black infants die *twice as often* as white infants.[87]†

America is the most dangerous place to be *pregnant*, with the highest maternal mortality rate of any first world country, of which deaths 60 percent are entirely clinically preventable by things as simple as taking the mother's blood pressure.[88] ‡

---

*   Compared to other high-income, industrialized countries, the United States experiences the highest rate of deaths otherwise preventable by timely access to medical care.

†   "Black infants in America are now more than twice as likely to die as white infants—11.3 per 1,000 Black babies, compared with 4.9 per 1,000 white babies, according to the most recent government data—a racial disparity that is actually wider than in 1850, 15 years before the end of slavery, when most Black women were considered chattel."

‡   And while Black, low-income, and rural patients are at the highest risk, pregnancy and childbirth complications threaten to kill pregnant people of every

America is the most dangerous place to be a child.[*]
America is the most dangerous place to be a woman.[89][†]
America is the most dangerous place to be gay.[90][‡]
America is the most dangerous place to be old.[91][§]
America is one of the most dangerous places to be disabled.[¶]

In 2017, life expectancy at birth fell for the first time in almost 30 years, by a tenth of a year.[92] There were 4 million people born that year. That's a theft of 400,000 years.

But a funny thing happens when you look at these statistics.[**] When you study them closely, you realize that all this danger only exists . . . if you're *poor.* Because rich people are exempt from all of these problems. Rich people have *exempted*

---

race, ethnicity, educational attainment, income level, or geographic area.

[*] A given child in the United States has a 70 percent greater chance of dying before they reach adulthood than other countries in the thirty-six-country Organisation for Economic Co-operation and Development (OECD). Over 600,000 children (roughly the population of Milwaukee, for context) have needlessly perished on American soil since 1961, who would not have died had they been born anywhere else in the developed world.

[†] Over 16 million women reported living in poverty in 2016. On average, they tend to have more healthcare needs than cis men (women are twice as likely to suffer from depression, for example), yet roughly one in four delay or forgo care due to cost.

[‡] AIDS, which disproportionately affects the LGBT population, has impacted the United States more than any other developed country.

[§] Among "high-need" older adults, a third of U.S. seniors skipped care because of costs, compared to only 2 percent for Sweden. A quarter of seniors reported concerns about having enough money to buy nutritious food, pay rent or bills, given their high medical costs. In France, the UK, Norway, and Sweden, by contrast, fewer than 5 percent of seniors said they struggled financially due to health costs.

[¶] OECD has maintained that the Social Security disability standard is among the strictest in the industrialized world because the majority of applicants are denied. Those who do qualify for benefits are the sickest of the sick, with multiple serious impairments or a terminal illness.

[**] You know precisely what I'm going to say. You feel it every second of your life. It is woven into the American fabric.

themselves from these problems. Men born in the wealthiest fifth of Americans get to live *15 years longer* than men born in the poorest fifth. Among women, that gap is 10 years.[93]

This has not happened on accident. America has chosen to refuse to recognize the essential dignity of being human. And in this refusal it has caused mass suffering. This is the terrible secret of American healthcare. This is the fundamental American illness. They're killing us and robbing our corpses to foot the bill. This is an act of *war*.

Enough.

PART II:

WHAT WE WANT

PART II: WHAT WE WANT

This big, stupid profit-driven multi-payer Rube Goldberg machine of American healthcare is failing us today and, left unchecked, will collapse tomorrow. So we—we who have been trapped in the quicksand of American health finance; we who have watched our families, friends, and neighborhoods be torn apart by the ravages of corporate greed; we who fear tomorrow—demand something more, and something better. We demand something that rejects that some people are born to suffer and instead offers a vision of hope and help for all people—that all may be treated as we wish our own children might be.

We now understand the general arrangement of private insurance, and we understand how it, by its very nature, is incapable of resolving the problems it has created. Private insurers know this too, and every time they're threatened, they bellow and wail about how any discussion of their great grift is an assault on consumer freedom. To them, "consumer freedom" is when we hope our employers let us choose from among a series of insurance plans that *might* cover us if we get very ill. "Consumer freedom" is our hope we never get fired or need to quit or ask our children to ration their insulin. They administer a game under this banner of "consumer freedom" that is rigged in their favor, and for three generations we've played it meekly—knowing we're getting robbed, but too afraid to throw the whole game out, rules and all.

No longer.

In this section of the book, I will illustrate that what we demand is a *federal universal single-payer*. I will walk through a definition of the program and what it contains. Since healthcare looms large over campaign season, we hear lots of confusing--named competitors to single-payer out there. They are lousy, each one of them, and I will explain why.

I just spent the first section of this book outlining how our current healthcare model works—and how it doesn't. It's a messy and loathsome thing, with thousands of lashing tongues and gnashing teeth; its complexity creates little dark corners in which lurk the deeper cruelties. What a staggering diversity of pain "consumer choice" has afforded us! We all can suffer at the hands of Aetna and Blue Cross and Humana in unique and personalized ways.*

While I don't think this complication is necessarily *intentional*, a healthcare model this labyrinthine is a healthcare model with plenty of opportunities to leech profit.† There are certainly people who benefit from this entire arrangement and are in no hurry to change it. Their profit almost directly correlates with our misery.

After a while this whole situation starts to warp the way you think. How couldn't it? Our lives are held hostage by the corporate transactions of insurance companies as we wait to learn whether they'll approve the procedures or medications we need to live the way we want. Or worse, we wait, captive, as deliberations we can't see and don't understand determine whether our insurers will pay for treatment we've *already* received—for which a denied claim could mean medical bankruptcy.

It's overwhelming. This big machine dominates you in body and spirit, and it's hard to shake it off. You get treated like

---

* So much for the power of the consumer "free market"

† We call this "innovation" in capitalism.

a captive for so long that you start to *believe* it—a kind of health insurance Stockholm syndrome. It happens to me, too: I've had enough denied claims that when another one comes in, my first instinct is to blame *myself* for seeking healthcare the "wrong" way, or not pushing against my doctors hard enough. We confuse paperwork and profit motives with the care we actually need to stay alive.

We've just absorbed the ideology of those who seek to profit from our illness. It's even infected our language. We call this whole thing "healthcare," but that's not right. At some point we confused the corporate transaction of *selling insurance* with *healthcare*. We confused the profit motives of companies with the care we need to stay alive. We've been led to believe that all of this has to be *hard*. It doesn't.

Providing healthcare—being a nurse, being a social worker, being a home-health aide, being a doctor—is hard. Our bodies are big bags of barely understandable goo that hurt all the time;[1] relieving their miseries is a difficult process. But paying for that care doesn't need to be difficult—not even on a national level. Paying for it is, honestly, rather simple.

In fact, the complexity of the *provision* of healthcare must not be used as an excuse to mask the simplicity of the *payment* for it—no matter what the people who make money from it insist. The bloated, impenetrable ACA was originally intended to massively subsidize private companies and hope they'd consider insuring sick people in exchange. Instead, it's being used to massively subsidize private companies *without* guaranteeing the insurance afterward. This is the natural consequence of compulsive compromise and the fetishization of incomprehensible "data-driven" policy. It is a murder at the hands of a legion of prissy policy people, a death by a thousand paper clips.

When these massive policies fall apart, it is not the policy nerds who find themselves unable to access healthcare. It is not the liberal compromise-worshipping think tanks* who learn their kid's surgery will put them into lifelong debt and spend evening after evening staring out the kitchen window into the night. If their skin isn't in the game, why play by their rules?

The insistence that healthcare finance must be obtuse, that we must be condemned to illness because of an untranslatable series of runes and glyphs accessible only to a specialized wonk class—that it just has to be *hard* and thus anything that isn't hard isn't a solution—is a kind of epistemic violence against us non-wonk humans.† It is a lack of ambition, disguised as pragmatism.

So let's start simple. Here's single-payer in one sentence: *we pool the money we already pay to insurance companies and use it to insure* everyone, *in full, with no cost-sharing.*

That's the long and short of it. Instead of privatizing risk pools, we make a single national risk pool and put everyone (*everyone*) in it. This pool is used to pay for everyone's healthcare: it is a *single* payer. This isn't science fiction, and it's hardly a novel idea—versions of single-payer exist all over the globe.

But what could that look like in the United States? Not all single-payer models are created equal, and not all universal healthcare models are rooted in a single payer. And if you can design a *good* single-payer model, you could certainly design a *bad* single-payer model. I'd like to walk through both—that is, I'd like to answer the questions, "What is single-payer" and "What *isn't* single-payer?"

---

*   At least, not the *executives* of the think tanks, who make sure they get paid even at the expense of their miserable, idealistic entry-level employees.

†   Sorry for using a nerdword. Let's define epistemic violence as harm caused by either the restriction of information from a person (e.g., that one needs to subscribe to an expensive journal and learn how to read specialist language to learn basic health policy) or the restriction of a kind of person from contributing to a broader discourse (e.g., school libraries refusing to stock Black history).

WHAT IS SINGLE-PAYER?

I wasn't being glib earlier. *Federal universal single-payer*, hereafter just "single-payer" or "single-payer healthcare,"* really is a pretty simple concept. Instead of subsidizing a bunch of relatively weak insurers and their fragmented customer bases and risk pools, each of which seeks to mitigate rising healthcare costs by avoiding taking care of unprofitable sick people, we have *one* publicly owned, publicly funded insurer with a mandate to cover, in full, *all* care for *all* people.

That phrase "all care for all people" isn't a slogan. It's a life-and-death necessity for an adequate healthcare program. Single-payer is often described as "Medicare for All," which is a helpful marketing device.† But it's inaccurate—for this real and robust single-payer program is a significant departure from how Medicare currently works in the United States. You may recall that Medicare has quite a bit of cost-sharing, out-of-pocket spending, and especially challenging drug and long-term–care costs (that harm both older people and people with disabilities or diseases).

Thus, a literal Medicare-for-all program is inadequate—instead, we demand an *improved* Medicare for all, which offers *comprehensive coverage, including medical, vision, dental, and long-term care‡ for all people in America, including noncitizens, that is free to receive with no cost-sharing.*

Here's how that looks in practice as a patient. Right now,

---

* FUSP has, for some reason, failed to really take America by storm as an acronym.

† Again—for some unknowable reason, people prefer to rally around M4A more than they do FUSP.

‡ The reiteration of long-term care is important. It's often treated like an "accessory" kind of healthcare, despite the fact that the aging Boomer population means it'll affect tens of millions of families in the coming decades.

if you go to the hospital, or you call a clinic to schedule an appointment, the first thing you're asked—sometimes even before your name—is who your insurer is. That's because providers are afraid of offering services, especially ones that are expensive to provide, without guarantee of reimbursement from an insurance company. Before we can even be considered for care, we must answer, "On whose dime?"

Under this single-payer model: You go to the local clinic or the hospital. Maybe you go to the one nearest your house, because you no longer need to navigate your insurance network. You go to the front desk, check in, wait for your name to be called, talk to the nurse, talk to the doctor, maybe get a prescription, and go home. Payment is never discussed—it doesn't need to be. We know who's paying for it: Medicare.

There's no good reason we can't live in the latter model instead of the first. There's no good reason you should work *against* your doctor—checking his or her every move to make sure it fits within your insurance plan, double-checking to make sure services you need are covered—and there's no good reason you are made to fear your bill if you fail. There's no good reason doctors have to spend half their day filling out forms to justify their work to insurance companies; there's no good reason nurses must spend over a quarter of their time adjudicating claims and seeking authorization for service from insurers.

There's no good reason for *any* of this. And so a single-payer system replaces your "no good reason" with "no longer." No longer will someone needing help be bound by maze-like "provider networks." No longer must you decide between food and medicine. No longer will your care, your partner's care, or the care of your children be decided by who your insurer is—the insurer is the single-payer. The insurer is Medicare. Go to the doctor and seek what you need.

HOW CAN WE AFFORD IT?

There are two answers to this question.

One, America—you, me, our insurance plans if we have them, the government—is *already* spending the money required to fund single-payer. We're just forced to use that money very stupidly, on bloated costs and corporate extortion. The insurance industry is just incompetent and unable to pay its share—Medicare is almost 33 percent more efficient than private insurance[2]—so it passes the costs to you.

In 2017, we spent about $3.5 trillion in national healthcare expenditures (NHE).[3] American public money pays the majority of those costs—the single-payer advocacy organization Physicians for a National Health Program argues that public money pays *two-thirds* of all NHE.[4] Whether through actual government healthcare spending—Medicare, Medicaid, the VA, etc.—or rewards to private corporations, the government, in one form or another, subsidizes the health insurance of almost every single insured person in the United States. We are literally subsidizing corporations—insurance companies, who get government subsidies, and our own employers, who get tax breaks—for selling us insurance we can't afford.

The remaining expenditures come from *out-of-pocket spending*—in a sense, an additional private tax you pay to insurers and healthcare corporations, in the form of premiums, deductibles, and co-pays.

On top of all that, we know that spending money through insurance companies isn't efficient. Insurers don't get good prices from providers, they don't focus on long-term health spending, and they hang on to some portion of the money passed through them to build offices, pay millions of dollars to their executives, and hoard profit. That's money nobody is using to take care of people.

Do you know what a pachinko machine is? They're really fun. You could think of them as Japanese slot machines.* Imagine a vertical pegboard with a bunch of little buckets at the bottom and dozens and dozens of pegs forming a kind of maze to reach them. To play, you drop a bouncy ball at the top of the board and watch it hit the pegs as it finds its random path toward the bottom. If it lands in a designated bucket, you get a prize. Naturally, the forces of air resistance and gravity will send most of your balls on wild and unpredictable journeys, and even if you know precisely where and how to place them, it's unlikely that they'll all end up in your preferred bucket.†

American health finance infrastructure is like dropping a bunch of quarters into a pachinko machine and only using ones that land in a certain bucket to pay our health costs. The rest sit in some private company's vault, or are used to pay inflated prices, or to deposit six-figure bonuses in an insurance CEO's savings account, or to lobby senators. If we were to use the money we're already spending *smarter*, in ways designed to address health costs instead of stripping off pieces to enrich men and women in suits, we'd be able to take care of more people. A *lot* more people.

So that's one reason single-payer is within our means. The other is that we frankly can't afford *not* to transition to single-payer. Rising healthcare costs are a problem in every country with some sort of national healthcare plan, but ours rise both the fastest and, led by unit costs (as described previously), the most unsustainably.

The current model offers no solutions except for national austerity—cutting Medicaid spending, basically—and increas-

---

*   Or as Plinko from *The Price Is Right*

†   There are now electronic pachinko machines, with extremely confusing rules and video-game-like interfaces, which I have spent approximately 10 US dollars playing with very little understanding of how.

ing the costs pushed onto patients. And patients can bend, and bend, but eventually they break. So long as private profit is put before public health, so long as the American multi-payer model persists, there is *no* way out of this hole. Though the problem is caused by large corporations seeking profit, the consequences for their actions will be borne by poor people, sick people, and the vulnerable.

But the rules are different for a single-payer healthcare model. A single-payer operates differently. It has tools by which it can mitigate rising costs without sacrificing its obligation to all of America's patients. One tool is the redirection of spending that otherwise would be used to fund insurers' administrative, profit, and marketing costs—a chunk of change very conservatively estimated at just under $400 billion a year.* Another is the de facto price-setting ability of a single payer. Remember how Medicare determines the fair price it's willing to pay for a given service and, because it covers 44 million members, hospitals accept it?† Scale that idea up to 330 million people. Negotiating with the maximal weight of all people in the nation who might choose to seek care, the single-payer can overnight reduce a lot of the price-gouging bloat in American healthcare unit costs while developing payment models that compensate providers justly. This is only the *beginning*.

It's so plain to see that a single-payer can bring medical costs down that even reactionary think tanks, or the Koch brothers, have to admit it. While I'm not a fan of dignifying the work of the wicked, their (accidental) agreement about single-payer's financial upsides is shocking. A paper pumped out of the bull-

---

*   ($383 billion) A less conservative, and perhaps more accurate, estimate calculates savings of approximately $504 billion, or half a trillion dollars, on annual administrative costs and overhead: https://annals.org/aim/fullarticle /2605414.

†   This advantage is the primary reason that Medicare costs have remained stable per person while private insurance costs have catapulted upward.

ishly pro-market Mercatus Center found that net health expenditures of an American single-payer program could save $2 trillion over the next decade compared to our current model's predicted rate of spending—and that's using some very optimistic projections of what the free market is capable of, and some very pessimistic ones of how a single-payer could work.[5] The Political Economy Research Institute at the University of Massachusetts, Amherst, pegs the 10-year savings of Bernie Sanders's bill in the Senate at $5.1 trillion.[6]

The real shock and awe of this Mercatus paper was the discovery that, while net health expenditures would decrease, the amount spent by the federal government would increase. This makes perfect sense when you remember that all spending is being done through the federal government instead of out of your pockets and mine. We're no longer paying taxes and subsidies and premiums and out-of-pocket spending—we make it simpler, more efficient, cheaper, and more humane for everyone. Bernie Sanders's team argues that a family of four who makes $40,000 annually spends about $5,700 on healthcare right now—in taxes, in insurance premiums, and in out-of-pocket costs. They project that under their single-payer plan (which we'll discuss more later), this amount would fall to under $500, replacing both existing Medicare and Medicaid taxes as well as insurance premiums.[7]*

The multi-payer model has had 40 years to figure this out. At every opportunity to do something good or even something useful, it has failed. Instead we have a hyperfragmented model that leaves people behind while increasing costs a projected 4–6 percent every year[8]—a growth rate *unbelievable* in any country with a comparable economy. This means that the $3.5 trillion we spent last year now will worm its way upward

---

* Of course, as we'll discuss later, Bernie's is not the only single-payer plan, nor should it be considered the be-all and end-all of single-payer, but it's a fine reference point.

over time—to $3.7 trillion, then $3.9 trillion, then, after a decade, to $4.5 or $4.7 trillion.

Granted, high healthcare spending isn't necessarily bad. America has a budget, it needs to go somewhere, and healthcare is both a very productive and high-return use of funds. If we've got all this money to spend, we *should* spend it on things like healthcare. God knows Congress signs blank checks for endless war or missiles every year, and health spending is certainly a much better (and higher-yield) use of public money than our permanent military operations across the globe. In a survey of European countries in 2013, every government dollar spent on healthcare saw a 400 percent return on investment—a fourfold increase in economic growth from spending driven by the initial government investment.* Contrast that with the almost 1,000 percent negative return on investment when public money is spent on defense, and you get a pretty good idea of why national healthcare expenditures aren't *inherently* a bad thing.[9]

But not all healthcare spending is the same. America spends twice as much per capita as its peer countries,[10] and we have very little to show for it. Sure, we have hospitals with art galleries inside of them, and a handful of insurance companies pulled in combined annual profits of $6 billion a few years ago (up 29 percent from the year prior),[11] but quality of care has stagnated or worsened for anyone who isn't extravagantly wealthy—and that's if you're lucky enough to be able to *afford* accessing healthcare in the first place. Almost half of low-income adults report going without care they need.[12] These massive expenditures are paid off the backs of people forced into poverty and debt for the crimes of being poor or sick.

---

* For example: increased government spending in healthcare goes to workers, who then go and buy things like food and toys, putting more money to their communities, which is also spent. Increased government spending in warfare goes to workers, sure, but it mostly goes to giant corporations and their investors.

So there's the technical answer: yes, we absolutely can afford it. There is no question among people who aren't being paid to throw grenades at the single-payer movement whether it can be afforded. But on a more visceral level, that question just feels a little backward to me. There is plenty of money to go around. There is an *unprecedented* amount of money to go around. We have so thoroughly ravaged the Earth—and I do mean the whole Earth—and taken, usually at gunpoint, its riches, that there are more than 2,000 billionaires in the United States. Eight of them have stolen more wealth than the combined financial value of half the people on the planet. It took me a long time to understand just *how much* a billion dollars is.

Here's a sense of scope: a million inches is fifteen and a half miles, or a little longer than the full length of Manhattan.* A billion inches is a round-trip flight between New York City and Beijing, with a layover somewhere.

There're weirdos out there walking around like vampires with a *billion* dollars and we've got entire communities where people grow up sick from toxic waste the state lets corporations dump in their backyards. The money to fund single-payer and *more* is out there—we just need to take back the money that has been stolen from us, instead of succumb to decades of brainwashing that teaches us we need to cut taxes on the hyper-rich and their pervert corporations so they can keep more of the money they make by hurting us.

So the question to me is not: can we afford this? It's not even: can we afford *not* to afford this? It's: this wealth has been

---

* For my non-Yankee readers, perhaps this extremely specific reference will help: one million inches is almost exactly the distance between Miron Bridge in Menasha, Wisconsin, and the St. Mary's parking lot in Oshkosh, if you walk over the old train track they turned into a bridge into Fritse Park, past the haunted house onto Main, then, take Commercial Avenue into the county roads alongside Lake Winnebago. Take Bowen south instead of following the highway past Cheatin Heart bar, and turn just past the radiator guy's house. The pizza place is pretty good if all this walking makes you hungry.

stolen from us; this wealth has been stolen from the people of the Earth; are we not *entitled* to collectively benefit from it? Otherwise—when the companies come whispering ruby promises of prosperity, when they drain our land and exhaust our labor, when they disappear to some other place where they can do the same thing cheaper—are we just to clutch our children and suffer silently through the night?

If we're spending this much on healthcare, if we're being ravaged and mined for cash, oughtn't we get our collective money's worth?

Whether you believe this money should come from taxing the 1 percent and their corporations their fair share, or whether you hold that the government* is the source of all its nation's money and can, to an extent, print money for federal programs,† or both—even without taxes, simply pooling together the money from deductibles, co-pays, premiums, and government spending is more than enough to fund single-payer—in fact, the amount you personally spend would *decrease*.[13]

One final note on the cost of single-payer. Single-payer advocates, including me, argue that single-payer will "cost less" than our total healthcare spending now. I think that's credible, and I believe it. But suppose the counterexample. What if, somehow, single-payer costs more money than what we're spending now?

Remember this equation from earlier in the book: healthcare spending is a function of healthcare costs multiplied by utilization.

Right now, we understand that we have artificially high costs, which result in artificially deflated utilization: hospitals and manufacturers and pharma companies charge exorbitant

---

*   Rather, "a government owning and controlling real resources, with an independent currency"

†   This is a view agreed upon by deeply conservative economist Alan Greenspan.

prices, and insurers can't, or don't want to, pay them, so they increase your co-pays and deductibles, and you therefore go to the doctor less.

It's entirely possible that a single-payer reverses this model: low costs but high utilization, to the point where we spend more money than we spend now. It is possible that our ability to access healthcare has been so thoroughly dammed, that we suffer from such a surfeit of clinical disorders and the extra-clinical disorders that cause them, that a great wave of patients will descend upon the hospitals and clinics to which they were previously denied access. And they will be met, in turn, their care determined not by their ability to pay but by their need.

But this is not a cause for concern. This is a cause for celebration. For it means that all America's people are freer in their bodies: free to live, free to work, free to care for their families, free to pursue that which makes them happy. It is a great unshackling of the American people.

That health economics is a hard science is a fantasy peddled by health economists. Even the greatest text in the field, *Pricing the Priceless* by Joseph Newhouse, is as much philosophy and theory as it is mathematics. Forecasting the utilization of healthcare is as precise as forecasting the weather. But I don't need to know what happens tomorrow to know what's happening today, and what's happening today is fucked. A complete reimagining of American health finance is needed. Any sufficiently wealthy nation owes its people the liberty of their own bodies. We can afford it, and therefore we must.

WHAT MIGHT IT LOOK LIKE?

You might wonder what a single-payer healthcare system could look like. Ultimately, that's a policy decision, and there's more to a good program than just its funding structure. I'm more interested in *power*—the stuff you and me are part of, the power of a popular movement that demands single-payer and, beyond it, health justice. But if I were called upon to design the implementation, I would consider these components as essential:

- **Comprehensive coverage, paid in full.** "All care for all people." Whatever care a person needs—medical, dental, mental, vision, reproductive, long-term care, and more—must be covered at no expense to the patient.

The way it is now, you walk into the doctor's office or the hospital and hope your insurance plan works there. No plan, no network, no healthcare. Need to see an endocrinologist for your diabetes or a cardiologist for your heart? If they're not in network, and sometimes if you didn't get a referral first, you can't see them—even if they're someone whom your doctor trusts and likes to work with.

Under a single-payer model, you walk into whatever office you want, see whichever doctor you want, and get whatever care you need, without having to pay anything out of pocket. This is *the* defining feature of what single-payer healthcare can be in America.

Traditionally, healthcare in America has been rationed according to race and one's ability to pay. Removing both these barriers to care permits the single-payer to give people what they need, want, and deserve. There are, and will be, instances in which demand outstrips supply of a medical good or service—organ transplants are a classic example. Single-payer models determine eligibility for care by "medical necessity": that is, does the person's medical provider believe the care is needed, and, if there is some unavoidable supply shortage, who needs it most? Fundamentally, I agree with the rule.

Much of the language around "medical necessity" exists to counteract a mythical person who will seek unnecessary care repeatedly. Perhaps this person gets recreational knee surgeries, taking up knee surgery slots that could be given to aging Boomers, members of the Green Bay Packers, or you. Perhaps this person is drug- or attention-seeking, and repeatedly checks into the ER seeking care they don't need. If you're a health economist, you fear and revile this person, because he brings up medical costs and promotes inefficient spending. If you're a morally upright person, you understand that this person *does* need medical care—just not the care they're seeking. They might need therapy, rehabilitation, or just help navigating the medical and welfare system to access the resources they need to stay out of the hospital. In this case, the single-payer must fund the employment of social workers required to help patients navigate their options for care with the warmth and empathy they deserve.

I would be careful with a strict definition of "medical necessity," however. I can think of three exceptions to this standard. First, I would exempt providers from clinical guidelines for care if they and their patient have a credible belief that such a deviation is best for the patient. Second, a specific pathway for people seeking trans healthcare needs to exist—otherwise, people seeking care would need a clinical diagnosis of some type of disorder ("gender dysphoria," for example) to get the healthcare they need. This is a kind of abrasive friction that results in some trans people dropping out of the healthcare system altogether. Third, people, especially people with disabilities, need a process for getting care they need that isn't strictly clinical—ASL classes for parents of Deaf children, for example, or accessible vehicles for people with mobility issues.

- **A single risk pool.** "All care for all people" means *all* care, of course, but also *all* people. This means the risk pool has to include poor people—and it absolutely must include rich people as well. Rich people are certain to demand the ability to "opt out" of contributing to the single-payer and purchase private insurance instead. This abuse of "consumer choice" language is not only insufficient, but actively dangerous. Rich people will find ways to buy their own private insurance plans, or pay for their own care directly, because they want luxury services and boutique care. If they do, and if there's no way to prevent it, whatever, fuck 'em—they just can't be permitted to do so in a way that undermines and saps the national risk pool.

We don't need to speculate about why not, because we've already seen this dynamic play out in South Africa. There, a basic universal insurance program exists, but people have the ability to decline to participate in it and instead spend in the private insurance market.* Private insurance usually charges significant premiums, but has access to private hospitals, nicer amenities, and other comforts and luxuries. If you're a wealthier person, you want these perks, so you pull out of the public insurance pool and purchase the private plan instead. Fewer enrollees means the public option has less room to bargain on prices—and because those enrollees are disproportionately poor, they tend to need more, and more expensive, healthcare.† Conversely, private insurers (because they have little bargaining power and a captive customer base) pay *extremely* high prices to a network of healthcare providers who refuse to work with the public payer.

As a result, 16 percent, or just under one-sixth of the population, spends just under *half* of South Africa's health expenditures. That 16 percent is wealthy, privately insured,

---

* South African president Cyril Ramaphosa announced a plan to create a universal risk pool and make national health insurance compulsory and universal in South Africa. As of February 2019, it is on its way to Parliament, and (from what South African papers I could find online) is expected to pass, despite fervent opposition from the private insurance industry. Sound familiar?

† We'll talk more about why this is, in the third part of the book.

and disproportionately white. By permitting private carve-outs from the national risk pool and national bargaining power, South Africa's healthcare model has virtually *reenacted apartheid* through market-driven healthcare finance.[14] We cannot permit similar splintered financing in America, lest we, too, re-perpetuate our historical denial of care for reasons of race and income.

- **Standards, payment, and administration at the federal level.** Standards for what care is covered have to be set at the federal level, and all payment must come from federal dollars. Medicaid shows us why: when states are permitted to determine what kind of care they cover, *and* when they're on the hook for the costs of that care, even a small economic slump can trigger state Medicaid programs to restrict services or find ways to recoup the costs from the patients.

This push-pull struggle of Medicaid incentives is carved into the bodies of people with disabilities. Think back to Steve and Kyle from the introduction of this book. Long-term care, particularly home health, is a good study—it's a matter of life and death for people who need it, and, because it's the kind of thing you tend to need for years and years, it's expensive to the state to provide it.*

This leads to sharp inequities in the provision of long-term care across the country. Richer states, effectively lobbied by disability rights organizations, offer care closer to humane while poorer states gut it. In Colorado, one of the more generous programs in the country, elderly or disabled people making less than $40,000 a year can receive home-health services without paying an additional premium. In Alabama, persons making less than $24,000 a year who have very few other assets (and limited spousal

---

* That home health lets people have the dignity of agency, and even pursue work they enjoy, is rarely factored into this cost equation.

income) face compulsory relocation into nursing homes, unless there happens to be a vacancy among the state's few thousand home-health placements. Sometimes people in Alabama need to divorce or leave their families so they can move to states like Colorado. But some horrors transcend state lines: in every state, Medicaid is permitted to *put a lien on your house—which accrues interest—*after you're in a long-term care facility for a few months.

This is the weakness of the Medicaid model and an argument for building a single-payer program out of the federally controlled Medicare. Weak state payers, like Medicaid programs, are vulnerable to bad actors and susceptible to the whims and fancies of ostensibly cost-sensitive local governments, who aren't always willing to fund essential programs if those programs run the risk of being expensive. This harms people who need those programs and cannot be part of any American implementation of a single-payer model. It must be the federal payer's responsibility to set comprehensive baseline benefits, negotiate costs, then pay for all of it. Let states have no incentive to avoid their responsibility, to turn their back on those who are sick.

- **Local implementation**. That's not to say that this should be an entirely federal program. Healthcare needs are local and there is value in local implementation of healthcare programs, even when those programs are paid federally. Across all America, healthcare needs look very different between states like Iowa and Texas. Across all Texas, healthcare needs look very different between cities like El Paso, McAllen, or Houston. Within a city like Houston, healthcare needs differ between Houston's majority Black, mostly poor Third Ward, and its excruciatingly posh, blindingly white River Oaks neighborhood just a few miles away. A federal agency simply can't be productive or proactive in adjusting for all these local needs.

There is precedent for a solution in existing Medicaid—the waiver program. Medicaid waivers let state agencies deviate from federal guidelines by adding, expanding, or substituting new programs for Medicaid enrollees, so long as they can prove that the new programs provide equal or greater care. There are programs all over the map—from financing holistic models of maternal health,[15] to funding home- and community-based care instead of institutional care for people with long-term medical needs, to programs that invest money in housing and food.[16] Like all systems, it's vulnerable to abuse, especially under Trump's Centers for Medicare and Medicaid Services (CMS) head Seema Verma and her red-eyed bloodlust for Medicaid work requirements, but at its best these waivers let states tailor care to the people who need it.

The immediate healthcare needs of 330 million people, whose cities and experiences are almost unimaginable in breadth, are far too nuanced for a singular federal entity to manage. The federal single-payer must guarantee payment for that care and set prices for treatment, but the local implementation of single-payer should have room for experimentation and customization at the state level—maybe even at the county level.

- **Budgeting tools.** Any single-payer model will have to guard itself against healthcare fraud and corporate abuse. Luckily, it will have many budgetary tools by which to do so. None of them are sufficient on their own, but in combination they can weave together like links in a suit of chain mail to protect our investments in our health and well-being:
  - Global budgeting: This is a fancy name for the advance determination of the national healthcare budget (e.g., "We're going to spend 3.5 trillion dollars this year"). This budget is then used to set baseline payment agreements for the year and

pay hospitals guaranteed blanket sums of money based on expected activity. If the single-payer looks at a hospital and determines it spent $30 million last year, it can predict that the hospital might need $33 million this year and guarantee that sum for an agreed-upon amount of work. This way the single-payer can pay hospitals fairly while minimizing the hospital's ability to rack up line items and gouge the government.

o   Restrictions on usage of single-payer money: that is, a single-payer can prohibit a hospital from using its payments to fund political activity, union-busting, marketing, or profit.

o   Different kinds of payment schemes for different kinds of providers, especially independent physicians or smaller clinics, depending on their patient loads and needs. Three common payment schemes are fee-for-service, bundled payment, or capitation models. Fee-for-service is a traditional line-item billing, where doctors tally up all the things they did and present an invoice. Bundled payment models offer a fixed amount, plus modifiers, per diagnosis (e.g., "an uncomplicated knee surgery will be reimbursed at X thousand dollars"). Capitation payments give doctors a set amount of money (plus modifiers for age and complexity) per patient, per month or year.

There's no one right tool for paying all doctors, so giving the single-payer the ability to rotate between a set of options for smaller providers keeps everyone happy while protecting public money.

★   ★   ★

When imagining what implementation of a single-payer system might look like in America, people tend to have some common questions. Let's address those as well:

What Happens to Existing Insurance Companies and Their Employees?

Supposing we don't just legislate them out of existence—which would be my dream scenario—existing insurance companies don't have to go, but they certainly can't stay here. A good single-payer plan prohibits the sale of insurance plans that compete with the public plan. Humana, Aetna, and friends might continue to sell supplemental luxury insurance plans to wealthy people (giving them, for example, access to the luxury suites at hospitals) or pivot into business ventures beyond health insurance—some of them will probably try to make money off single-payer by acquiring healthcare providers.* I'd prefer a more dramatic option: though I don't like gilding the pockets of the wealthy, the cost to nationalize the health insurance industry during the negotiations of the Affordable Care Act was under a quarter trillion dollars, or a thirteenth of current national healthcare expenditures.[17] That's without question a smart (and cost-efficient) investment; plus, we get the technology and infrastructure these companies have developed.†

---

*   I don't know if there's a legal way to prevent them from doing so, but if there is, I'm for it.

†   This is most exciting because it means we might finally have a standardized data format and transfer method for healthcare data. Electronic health records were made by sequestered private companies and the result is a total libertarian wasteland. A single, standardized method of data input and transfer would both be a blessing upon any exasperated doc and reduce the significant hassle and error rate of our current byzantine infrastructure.

But I am not interested in comforting the companies; I care about people. We can't leave employees of insurance companies behind because they work in a nationalized industry. Luckily, we're not going to. One of the greatest strengths of both Pramila Jayapal's House bill and Bernie Sanders's Senate bill are their massive allocations for the retraining and replacement of workers in the insurance industry. This should be the norm in all future discussions of single-payer. But what does that mean?

The People's Policy Project (PPP) posits that there are approximately 2.6 million people who work in the health insurance sector. (That sounds like a lot, and it is, but for comparison—across all industries, approximately that many people are laid off or otherwise leave their jobs every 54 days.)[18] We seek to remove the exploitative industry of private insurance and create a more perfect public insurer, and many of these jobs will need to exist under a single-payer: someone will need to write the code, process the claims, and analyze the data that undergirds the operations of insurance.

Beyond the rows of computer touchers, many people employed in insurance are customer support staff working in a call center, or nurses who are hired to dispute bills with other nurses in hospitals. Much of the work of insurance companies boils down to nurses in one high-rise office building arguing with other nurses in different high-rise office suites about how much care a patient *really* needs. If you work at an insurance company, chances are your job is to identify the bare minimum of care you're required to cover, and then cover only that—fundamentally, your job is to talk to people on the phone and give them less care than they might want. This is the labor of insurance.

But single-payer healthcare doesn't erase jobs or make them redundant. If it wants to get its work done, a single payer has to *create* jobs. A *lot* of jobs. Meaningful jobs.

Let me give you an example. There's a model of Medicaid

clinic known as a *medical-legal partnership*. It's fantastic. It understands that a person's health is dependent upon things that happen way outside of the doctor's office.

Here's how one medical-legal partnership in heavily segregated Boston works. Someone walks in with their kid. Their kid is having trouble breathing. Behind the desk is a social worker, who listens to the parent, takes comprehensive notes, communicates them to medical staff, then escorts the parent and child to a clinic room. A nurse or doctor enters, and they perform a checkup—yup, the kid has asthma; let's get her a prescription for an inhaler.

But that's not where it stops. Because the social worker knows that asthma in kids is often caused by housing conditions, and since this is a Medicaid clinic, it's likely that the family's housing might be substandard. *What's your home like?* the social worker asks. *Well, we're poor*, replies the parent. *We live in a slum. We've got water in the ceiling and mold in the walls.*

The social worker knows this kind of living condition absolutely causes asthma. And, in fact, they know that there are civil and legal protections against it. There are a *lot* of civil protections against things that make you sick. But you only have access to these protections if you can afford to hire a lawyer—or if you have the free time and fluency to represent yourself.

The social worker brings the patient another door down and brings in a lawyer, or a law student operating under a lawyer's purview. They write a letter threatening to sue the patient's landlord and send it off. Within a month, the water and mold are cleaned up.

This social worker is one face of the labor of single-payer. A single payer *has* to invest in these kinds of jobs—they bring long-term costs way, way down. And what's their job, ultimately? To take a person who needs care and find all the possible kinds of care to which they are entitled. Isn't that just an inversion of the responsibilities of the jobs offered to us by private insurance? Wouldn't it be so much nicer to let people use their professional skills in service of their communities, instead of corporate profit they'll never touch?

This obviously does not accommodate all workers in the insurance industry, and I can't claim to have a perfect jobs-transition plan in my back pocket. I only mean to point out that there's a lot of *work* in the service of operating a single-payer program—kinds of creative, compassionate work that private enterprise is just unable to value—work that respects obligations to both insurance workers and the broader healthcare needs of the American people.

Besides, unyielding suffering has been wrought upon America in the shadows of these corporations I propose shuttering. Because of them, tens of millions of people are without insurance, while tens of millions more are underinsured. Do we let these people die because we wish to preserve an industry? No. Let us find the jobs they need, let us comfort all the afflicted, and let us forever turn our back on our destroyed insurer Sodom.

Is This a Gradual Transition Process or Does It Just Happen Overnight? What About My Current Insurance Plan?

Fears of dramatic disruptions in insurance are predicated in a misconception that the current American model is smooth and continuous. Far from it: we currently have a deeply disruptive health insurance enrollment process. If you have employer-sponsored insurance, every year your plan ends and you have to pick a new one from a list.* To make that list, your HR de-

---

* It's more common for a group plan's benefit year to sync with the calendar year (e.g., January 1 to December 31). However, employers can align their insurance plans on some other arbitrary year designation (for example, May 1 to April 30).

partment has to negotiate with insurance companies to figure out which plans they're going to offer, and how much your boss is willing to contribute. Unless you're particularly lucky or wealthy, that list is extremely complicated, and all the good options are even *more* expensive than they were last year—and that's before the deductible of thousands of dollars.

If you don't have employer insurance, or if you lose your job at Christmastime layoffs, you're left to navigate either your state exchange website or healthcare.gov, which had so lousy a launch that even the venerable Big Dog T-shirt brand made fun of it.* There, the site attempts to guess your subsidy amount by asking for your prior year income—unhelpful if you have sporadic, irregular income, or if you just lost your job. If your income changes over the course of the year and it's not properly recorded, you might find yourself *retroactively ineligible* for insurance for care you've already received!

Enrolling everyone in a single-payer program is going to be a lot of work, but compared to our current mess, its implementation can be a relative breeze.† There's nothing too disruptive about enacting single-payer all at once at the end of a year—virtually anything would be less disruptive than what we have now.

Each year, millions of Americans enroll in Medicare as it is. This should be a simple process—and at one time, it was—but

---

* The shirt showed one of the namesake "Big Dogs" sitting in front of a computer that displayed the words *healthcare.goof*. In the background, in large letters, *CAN'T FIX STUPID*, a Big Dog catchphrase. This is a devastating and, frankly, very legitimate takedown.

† I'm interested primarily (for the purposes of this book) in the complexity of implementing single-payer from an enrollee's perspective. On the back end—of course, developing single-payer requires substantial expansion of current enrollment and data-capture capability, but since no premiums are being assessed nor payments received, and since we're no longer operating on the arbitrary business timelines of Open Enrollment, this seems like an eminently solvable project. We just can't use the contractor (or contracting process) that fucked up healthcare.gov so bad.

it has been made complex with Part B and Part D premiums and Medicare Advantage choices made tempting by Medicare's weaknesses. All these complexities are created not by some inherent characteristic of Medicare but by its intentional whittling down in favor of private corporate interests.

So make it a simple process again. Fill out a form in person, on the phone, or online, and get a benefits card on the spot, with an official one in the mail. Have a final Open Enrollment–style period in the last few months of the year, in which everyone enrolls in Medicare instead of private insurance. If you miss the deadline, you just enroll when you can and get retroactive care. To ease the burden on Medicare's servers, we could stagger enrollment period start dates over the course of the year, by birthday or by SSN. Since there's no need to lock in enrollees by a certain deadline for the benefit of private insurance companies, there's quite a bit of flexibility. Providers will know they're guaranteed payment for the services they provide, so there's no risk of being turned away at the door, even if a person's enrollment is held up.

If HHS were to determine that single-payer should be phased in more gradually, or if political pressure from the insurance lobbies wins out and they demand breathing room, that's possible too. Year One could give emergency care to all Americans, offer single-payer to all current Medicare and Medicaid enrollees, plus people under age 26. (This way the risk pool is a little more balanced, since the under-26 crowd is much less likely to need extensive healthcare.) The next year, expand it to people under 35 and over 55. The next year, all in.

This slow rollout is clearly suboptimal—it leaves people who desperately need healthcare out on a limb for the convenience of the private market, while giving insurance companies preferential treatment in their risk pools. I include it here only to show that there're multiple ways to transition to single-payer. We're hardly exploring new territory here: questions of "How do I enroll millions of people on an insurance plan?" have existing answers worldwide.

What about a "Socialized Medicine" Model, Like What the UK Has in the National Health Service (NHS)?

An American NHS, or the full nationalization of both health finance and health provision (that is, a situation in which the government is the payer, and the owner of the hospitals, clinics, etc. where you would go to receive care), would be fine by me. However, I do not think single-payer is necessarily a "lesser" option. It does not lead to worse outcomes: per the OECD, outcomes in countries with single-payer rival and occasionally exceed those of the UK.[19] It does not in and of itself remove profit from healthcare—there is still a complicated healthcare market and issues of medical grift and fraud in the UK. I think single-payer is eminently more winnable than an American NHS in America, since it focuses primarily on insurance companies, who are widely reviled by American voters. Taking over one's doctor, or one's hospital, is a harder sell. But most importantly, I believe public control over health finance gives us the tools to realize something more and better: democratic control of the things that affect our life and health. We'll discuss this more in Part 3.

How Are the Bills in Congress?

I am happy to announce that Representative Pramila Jayapal's (D-WA) bill satisfies all the requirements of single-payer I have outlined in this book. It is an astonishingly strong piece of healthcare legislation. Senator Bernie Sanders's (I-VT) 2019 "Medicare for All" bill solves several of the problems surrounding long-term care in this 2018 bill and is also, as of this writing, a bill which meets my criteria for a single-payer program.

Single-payer is a simple program that is affordable, necessary, and moral. By and large, you and me and the people we know understand we're being hosed by the insurance industry, and demand relief. But we must beware of those out there trying to co-opt this energy and funnel it into programs that ultimately benefit the same corporations that are hurting you in the first place. That's where the bills that aren't Sanders's or Jayapal's come in. Let's talk about those programs.

WHAT ISN'T SINGLE-PAYER?

Talking about healthcare in America today feels different than talking about it even in 2013. Though the implementation (and desecration) of the ACA slowed the wheels of the machine, more and more of us are being crushed by healthcare costs—while we see corporate profits skyrocket. It's plain to see that this just isn't right, and accordingly there's been a surge of interest in the single-payer, or "Medicare for All," movement—hell, that's the reason this book is being written when it is. At the time of writing, 70 percent of people nationwide indicated they were in favor of "Medicare for All."[20]* That rules.

---

* Naysayers argue that people who like single-payer decide they don't like it when asked about paying taxes. They neglect to mention that this support returns when people are reminded it would guarantee all care for everyone they know.

Unfortunately, health policy can get pretty complicated, and most well-adjusted people would generally prefer to spend their time, like, playing with their kids or going mudding or illegally downloading a video of one of the greatest wrestling matches of all time* than learning the nitty-gritty about American health finance. In this understandable confusion dwells a lot of potential for misinformation.

Fundamentally, single-payer requires reallocating a lot of money in the healthcare industry from corporate profit and CEO salaries toward taking care of people. There are many people, mostly people in D.C., who are very interested in catching the spirit of the popular health reform movement but also preserving the status quo of massive corporate profits. They are utterly convinced that only their "pragmatic" plans of more aggressively subsidizing private companies will make things better, and they convince themselves that their fancy-lad pedigrees mean they've got the whole thing figured out. For some reason, these people are listened to and even given great sums of money. They spend this money to hire consultants to tell them how to shift the momentum of the "single-payer" movement toward a more corporate-friendly solution.[21] Some of these people are the Democratic majority leader.[22] Here are some things to know so that you don't fall for it.

First: nomenclature. It's worth noting that "single-payer" and "universal healthcare" get bandied about as if they were synonyms. "Universal healthcare" and, even worse, "universal *coverage*" are, in America, nothingwords used to confuse you.

"Universal healthcare" means that everyone can get healthcare—nothing more. It does not imply any particular financ-

---

*   Randy "Macho Man" Savage v. Ricky "The Dragon" Steamboat at Wrestlemania III. Not the greatest match of all time, not even the greatest match of Steamboat's career (that would be his series against Flair in NWA), but without a doubt a deeply great match, and one that was so precisely written that it's accessible to people who don't think they like wrestling.

ing model or structure. It once referred to what we now call a federal single-payer program, but it has been diluted over the past few decades to mean very little on its own. It could mean anything from "federal universal single-payer" to just reimbursing preventive medicine and nothing more.

"Universal coverage" or "universal access" usually means "everyone should be able to purchase an insurance plan, and if someone isn't able to purchase a plan, we should spend a lot of public money subsidizing the insurance company." This in no way handles the problem of escalating costs, and (not surprisingly) compelling people to purchase insurance plans from private companies does nothing to address the actual structural problems of healthcare in this country. The "universal access to healthcare" idealized is more specifically universal access to *purchasing* insurance plans. By this standard—I technically have unfettered access to purchasing a Ferrari (or even another 2002 Honda CR-V), but access alone sure as hell ain't gonna get me behind the wheel.

Here are some other things that are not single-payer:

STATE-BASED SINGLE-PAYER, À LA "HEALTHY CALIFORNIA"

When pressured about single-payer, many powerful federal-level politicians avoid the question by indicating they'd like to see a state-driven solution. (They usually then cite Supreme Court justice Louis Brandeis and say something about states being the "laboratories of democracy.") This is an inappropriate solution, and they know it. States are *inadequate* to the task of single-payer.

There are several technical and logistical reasons why this is the case. First, the technical: if a state were to pass single-payer, it would need federal approval from all three branches of government. The executive branch would need to approve the state's Medicaid and Medicare waivers to adjust its allocation of federal funds to the state payer—under Trump (and his

Health and Human Services [HHS] secretary, former pharma exec Alex Azar, and *especially* under CMS chief Seema Verma, who led Indiana's path to gutting Medicaid and privatizing the scraps),* this is unlikely. Congress would need to pass a bill exempting the state from the Employment Retirement Income Security Act of 1974 (ERISA), the federal laws that govern self-insured employer-based plans.† They would not. Lastly, there would be the inevitable Supreme Court case, and there's a decent argument that this is a type of interstate commerce, which states aren't constitutionally permitted to regulate.

If these were to somehow be avoided, there are logistical roadblocks, primarily around spending. Unlike the federal government, states aren't allowed to "deficit-spend" (they can only spend from the revenue they receive, instead of incurring a debt). So the single-payer would need to be paid in full every year, probably through a consolidated tax on employers and employees. But healthcare spending is "countercyclical"—that is, you have more healthcare costs when the economy is down (for a lot of reasons, including the simple fact that being unemployed is stressful, and stress makes you sick)—so if you're a state single-payer program, and a recession hits, you're spending more on healthcare costs than what you're getting in. Now you're in a pickle. Another thing states don't have in common with the federal government is that they can't just reallocate funds from their infinite war programs or other cash-sinks, so they'd need to either cut from the healthcare program or pull

---

*   If the overwhelming, shameless, actively harmful grift of these hucksters—and the fact that they'll probably never be held accountable for a thing in their lives—disturbs you, be comforted in the knowledge that they are most certainly going to hell.

†   ERISA is a fascinating and very opaque law that has, not by original intent but by modern interpretation, handcuffed states that want to more aggressively regulate healthcare in their state. It's not possible to even create a state-sponsored resource pool for insurers (like a database of how much different procedures cost), because self-insured plans can't be required to participate.

dollars from other programs like schools or infrastructure.* Not good. Maybe it's possible that New York and California have the budget space necessary to fund a single-payer program in their state, or a buffer of state tourism revenue to protect against recession, but I'm skeptical.

I have to reckon that the powerful national figures who push for "state-based solutions" to the healthcare crisis are just shirking their responsibility to confront the same powerful donor class who profits from our market-based problem in the first place. If and when a state single-payer program fails, they'll point to it and say, "Oh, it didn't work in such-and-such a state; therefore, it can't work federally"—even though they know (and now you know) that state and federal single-payers are entirely different programs. I am therefore less inclined to encourage people to agitate for "Healthy State" state-based single-payer programs when the projected upside is minimal and the downside could be catastrophic. There are real programs—social housing programs, programs to get people out of prison, felon voting rights, education funding, and a constellation of infinite others—that can be won in your home state with its own resources to relieve the misery of the people surrounding you—and you can win them in a way that also builds a broader movement for single-payer healthcare. We'll discuss some of the ways these movements converge in Part Three of this book.

MEDICARE ADVANTAGE

There are also movements to expand the Medicare Advantage program beyond the current Medicare population. We spoke earlier about Medicare Advantage and how it's been given privileges over regular Medicare just so private companies can

---

* Or, as in Wisconsin, all three.

profit. This is fundamentally why any Medicare Advantage program is inadequate. But its poison runs deeper.

Medicare Advantage is a pretty lousy deal for everyone: it's bad for patients: it sings sweetly to you until you need to use it, when it becomes as byzantine and repressive as the worst non-Medicare private insurance plan (in fact, becoming ill or getting injured is a strong predictor of switching away from Medicare Advantage). It's bad for providers: it creates waterfalls of paperwork, delays in authorizations, and lower reimbursements than normal Medicare. It's bad for the public: it opens us up to massive cases of corporate (always corporate, never personal) fraud and abuse. And it's just generally bad: it is an exercise of an ideology utterly opposed to public investment in public wellbeing and seeks to siphon off public money into private coffers by any means necessary. Despite this, Medicare Advantage is enthusiastically championed by CMS itself while private insurers race to gobble up more and more customers. In 2019, they counted 20 million Medicare benificiaries enrolled in the private option.[23]

Except here's the thing—there's no money in insuring sick people. Definitionally, it's only profitable to insure people who don't need insurance—unless you're getting bailed out by someone else's money. So these plans need to do three things if they want to turn a profit: draw in inexpensive customers (hook 'em), restrict the amount they spend on providing insurance (cook 'em), and find a way to get bailed out by the feds afterward (crook 'em). We'll take each in turn.

1. Hook 'em: Privileges and Treats

Medicare Advantage plans are regulated in such a way that customers who use Part C are given special privileges over users of traditional Medicare. Most importantly, there's an out-of-pocket cap—which limits how much a customer can be made to spend in copays and cost-sharing, and which should be the norm for all Medicare plans. (You might once again suspect that traditional Medicare is kept flawed to make Advantage seem superior.)

Then there're the perks. Private Medicare wants to find ways to draw in mostly healthy patients to stay profitable. They're allowed to offer all kinds of basic dignities—like bundled vision and dental care—and shiny perks, like free Fitbits, Silver Sneakers exercise programs, and comped Lyft rides to the doctor's office and other shit.

These are good things. People should have them. I just think traditional Medicare should be allowed to offer them as well, instead of reserving them for the private sector. It's cosmically unfair, and by this own-goal unfairness the austerity movement tilts at the public Medicare program with big mole claws, eager to hollow it out and hoard the spoils.

2. Cook 'em: Restriction

Fitbit or no, you just can't dance away from the fundamental law of insurance: you can't really profit from paying for the healthcare of people who need a lot of healthcare. Medicare Advantage is great, until you really need to use it. Under the pretense of caring about "provider quality" or "care coordination"—real problems which can be addressed without throwing patients under the bus—Medicare Advantage makes it as difficult to seek healthcare as it was when you had employer-sponsored insurance.

Just like ESI, private Medicare plans have networks—narrow lists of providers you're allowed to see, at risk of major financial penalty. So you have to hope that your plan includes the doctors you like, or the doctors who work near you—if you're mobility-impaired, or in a nursing home, or just not able to travel very easy, you're hosed. Should have read all the confusing enrollment literature more closely.

Once you're able to actually get to a doctor, you're not out of the woods yet. People with complicated medical needs find themselves trapped in prior authorization hell—where they need to wait days or weeks to obtain insurer permission to get care like advanced CT scans (for which they bill the patient up to $300 a scan, compared to around $50–$75 under traditional Medicare). If you have complex medical needs, you can be stuck waiting and waiting and waiting, even when your oncologist needs to plan further treatment.

3. Crook 'em: Risk Adjustment

In theory, Medicare Advantage companies profit by being so good at narrowing networks, finding the best providers, and coordinating care, that they just happen to spend less than they take in. In reality, there's risk adjustment

Imagine a horrible scenario in which a patient with a lot of medical needs chooses Aetna's Medicare Advantage plan and then gets chemotherapy, several surgeries, and some extensive inpatient hospitalizations—imagine how expensive that would be! There's simply no way Aetna would break even on their allotment of public money for this patient. Hence, risk adjustment: a complex subsidy program designed to offset the risk that a patient needs to use the insurance they purchase. At the beginning of the insurance year, Medicare looks at the aggregate patient pool of Aetna, or any other Medicare Advantage insurer—patient ages, genders, and health status profiles. Based on this composition, Medicare offers a benchmark amount it is willing to pay Aetna for providing insurance. If Aetna thinks it can insure the population for less, it keeps the difference and can use that projected surplus on perks, treats, and profit.

If it turns out that a patient is sicker than Medicare guessed they would be when setting the benchmark, the government pays the private insurer a bonus to compensate for it, usually in the range of a few thousand dollars.[24]

These determinations of illness and their resulting insurer bonuses are made using diagnoses on a patient's medical records. Now, these medical records have two purposes: tracking patient status, and bringing in cash. Aetna and friends are thus interested in making sure every possible diagnosis that can be on those records gets on those records, regardless of whether it's a necessary or even true diagnosis. This is known as upcharting, and Medicare Advantage insurers are more interested in the data-heavy business of upcharting than the business of insurance.

An example: a doctor might see a patient and note that their potassium levels are low. Not catastrophically low, just a little low. These levels can vary from time to time, and so the doctor decides not to make a formal diagnosis or begin medications—a normal, standard thing in the course of a relationship between a patient and their doctor. The doctor decides not to diagnose the patient with hypokalemia and moves on. That's not good enough for Aetna. Aetna really wants that hypokalemia diagnosis, and that sweet risk-adjustment money—so it sends the patient back to a doctor with whom it has a prior agreement to chart as much as possible. The diagnosis is made. (Perhaps the second doctor works at a hospital which sells an upcharting program to Medicare Advantage insurers, and which thus pressures its doctors to diagnose everything whenever possible—or else face an onslaught of curious calls from the billing department.)

Finally, efficient healthcare!

A 2017 allegation from the Justice Department, dismissed under the Trump administration, claims that one single insurer, UnitedHealth, used its Medicare Advantage program to defraud the public of 3 billion dollars between 2010 and 2015. Former UnitedHealth finance director Benjamin Poehling agrees: he is the whistleblower at the center of the case.[25]

It is alleged that UnitedHealth did this in two ways: one, it identified diagnoses it thought it might be able to get approved, and pressured doctors to review a selected patient for them (upcharting); two, at the end of the insurance year, it did not delete diagnoses that were inaccurate or out-of-date.

Think about the scale involved here. UnitedHealth has about five million people enrolled in its Medicare Advantage program—getting an upgraded Medicare risk profile for just 4 percent of them would bring in an additional $600 million in public money a year.

This kind of billing fraud is extremely common. Dialysis giant DaVita agreed to a $270 million settlement just a few years ago.[26] Hell, UnitedHealth got busted doing the same thing in 2009, through its health analytics subsidiary Ingenix, which is also named in the current suit.* Whenever we hand over Medicare to private companies, they rip us off for billions and billions of dollars. The money we give is given at the expense of the American public, and it's money that's stolen from rural hospitals, public schools, or infrastructure. Medicare Advantage is a theft from the future of America.

Not great.

---

* Ingenix was led by Andy Slavitt, who went on to be President Obama's CMS chief. He is now behind the United States of Care, a think tank that seeks to put "healthcare over politics." Yet the man behind the largest Medicare Advantage fraud cases in history balks at any reform that actually addresses the material problems of the people he claims to care about. Whatever, dude.

MEDICARE EXTRA FOR ALL/MEDICARE FOR AMERICA/
THE PUBLIC OPTION

In February 2018, the center-left think tank Center for American Progress (CAP) released a "healthcare plan" called "Medicare Extra for All."* Medicare Extra for All (what a clownish name!) is a version of the *public option*—basically, a publicly run insurer that "competes" against private insurance companies.[27] Employers can choose Medicare Extra if they want to, anybody under 65 with employer insurance can enroll in it (while, of course, paying means-tested premiums for the privilege), and eventually it can be rolled out to replace Medicaid.

It is an attempt to try the ACA again, but a little bigger. This is admirable, but it doesn't address the underlying issues of American healthcare; it neither removes the fissures created by a system of separate and self-interested payers, nor does it help the people trapped between them. It maintains a standard of means-testing, or rationing by income, that has soured the ACA for millions of people.

Medicare Extra is still very much a *tweak*. It looks at the devastating problems in American healthcare—a broken machine, a fragmented insurance model, runaway costs, and the utter dehumanization of poor people and people who are sick—and instead of recognizing them as harmful structures to be destroyed, it hopes to *play nice* with them.

This represents the worst kind of bland centrist thinking: that the things causing the worst problems in America—health inequity, the sprawling carceral state, ecological disaster, structural homelessness—are just beyond our control and therefore not worth addressing directly. To this lazy, compla-

---

* You may be familiar with it as "Medicare for America," a bill proposed by two Democratic congresspeople and championed by former Texan congressman and Dem presidential hopeful Robert O'Rourke.

cent strain of thought, they must be accepted as givens to be avoided or mitigated. A band of wild horses stampedes across America and, according to CAP, we must appease them with subsidies and little bits of apple instead of bridling them and driving them away.

Then, of course, there is the more cynical reason CAP and other centrists advance such tepid, useless policy: they actively benefit from the donations of the insurance industry and hope to see its continuation. When meeting with Blue Cross executives, an aide to Democratic House Majority Leader Nancy Pelosi assured the insurance titans "not to worry" about single-payer, before asking for their financial and institutional support.[28] These organizations invoke the language surrounding the single-payer movement but neuter the policies to keep corporations happy. It is imperative that we understand and reject them.

THE "BUY-INS"

Other public option–style plans worth mentioning are the Medicare and Medicaid "buy-in" plans. Medicaid buy-in is what it says it is: people who would otherwise not qualify for Medicaid can purchase Medicaid as if it were a plan on the marketplace. Because Medicaid is different in each state, the robustness of your "public option" for health insurance coverage would be contingent on your zip code. Medicaid reimbursement for providers can be abysmal, and doctors tend to have to work harder to care for the poor, the sick, and the marginalized. Accordingly, there are in many areas a dearth of providers who are willing to accept Medicaid patients. Depending on where you live, Medicaid buy-in means you could be spending a decent chunk of change so that you can theoretically have "coverage" in the form of an insurance plan that many doctors won't take.

Medicare buy-in is similar to Medicaid buy-in, but instead it is the Medicare brand repackaged and brought to market. Medicare would ostensibly function as another ACA exchange plan option, with 10 essential health benefits and cost-sharing based on metal tiering (bronze, silver, etc.).

This sucks, basically. When we demand "Medicare for All," we don't mean "Medicare as it exists now." And for good reason. Medicare buy-in would cover 70–80 percent of your medical costs and push the rest back to you. Proponents would say that this is pragmatic, because it saves money by skimping on the full cost of care. Of course, this plan doesn't do anything about the skyrocketing costs of actual treatments and is of little use to you, the patient.

The overarching structure and vision of these buy-in plans reflect a near obsession with the status quo, an insistence on the hegemonic domination of employers and insurance companies on the health and well-being of people. These technocratic nerds have adopted a shared narrow-sightedness, unable to think beyond "what is": they never consider, for example, that this employer dominance was a historical accident, and that the suffering it inflicts is, in a sense, a slow-burning casualty of the second World War, not a divine mandate.

ARBITRARY EUROPEAN COUNTRIES

You might hear that other countries have achieved universal healthcare without a single-payer model. This is accurate. But their models could not be transferred to the United States.

The healthcare exchanges of the ACA were modeled off those in the Netherlands and Switzerland, two countries who have achieved so-called "universal coverage." Both countries rely on health insurance markets of individual plans offered by private insurers. To ensure enrollment, they have insurance mandates (punishments for not buying insurance) similar to the much-loathed ACA individual mandate. They provide premium subsidies for low-income folks, standardize benefits packages to ensure a minimum level of insurance plan quality, and use community ratings for premiums, meaning insurers in a given geographical region must sell a given policy to everyone, irrespective of health status, for the same premium. If this sounds familiar to you, it should—these are all the same tricks that the ACA employed in an effort to integrate good patient health outcomes into the ways and means of profit-hungry payers and providers. And as I'm sure you remember from Part 1 of this book, or perhaps your own life, it's not working.

These European insurance markets are rooted in the ideas of economist Alain Enthoven and his principles of managed competition. In theory, by the magical regulatory power of the free market, competition among payers and providers would contain costs. Providers who offer poorer-quality services or who demand expensive prices will have to either improve care quality, reduce their rates, or both. The theory of managed competition takes for granted the idea that patients and payers will somehow have the ability to differentiate between higher- and lower-quality services. Knowledgeable consumers will choose to "shop" elsewhere, and providers that don't cater to the demands of the free market will be forced to shutter their businesses.

But this idea, like the ideas of most economists, is based on pseudo-realities and wild presuppositions that don't reflect reality as we all know it to be.* As the markets in Netherlands and Switzerland clearly indicate, competitive insurance markets alone are not enough to bend the cost curve.

In Switzerland, the hospital sector is the main driver of rising healthcare costs, most likely because their health reforms

---

* I trust the magical worlds of Wizards of the Coast more than I trust the models of most economists.

have focused solely on insurance purchasing. Because the Swiss have not regulated contracting between insurers and hospital providers, costs continue to spiral out of control as providers demand high prices for services that might be superfluous or of poor quality. Even in spite of its insurance market regulations, most Swiss insurance plans are woefully inadequate for enrollees. Almost 90 percent of Switzerland's insured population is forced to purchase supplemental insurance on top of their main insurance plans to cover the dental and other services that their primary insurer refuses to provide.[29] Supplemental plans, in both the Netherlands and Switzerland, need not abide by some of the most crucial consumer protections baked into their respective primary healthcare markets. These plans can, for example, reject applicants and engage in risk-rating to keep their costs down. The many different insurance plans on the Swiss market foster confusion, or even fear; there are concerns that if their supplemental and primary plans are offered by different companies, an illness could cause supplemental plan premiums to skyrocket. And in the Netherlands, insurers have been known to risk-select by setting higher premiums for supplemental policies for people they believe to be riskier to insure or with some known illnesses.

As Dutch and Swiss citizens struggled to make ends meet during the peak of the recession, many people found themselves unable to afford insurance premiums. Both governments recognized this as a problem and decided to come to the aid . . . of the companies. Insurance companies were permitted to cut off coverage for defaulters, while the number of defaulters only rose, even among those who received subsidies. It's a big, stupid mess.

*   *   *

None of this is good enough. All these programs—from Medicare buy-ins to the Dutch model—might be better for some people than what we have in America, but they continue to leave behind those people who we are *already* leaving behind. They are structurally incapable of solving the problems that have torn this country apart. They are lesser measures. They are *compromises*.

These incremental half-measures are revolting to me. We suffer within a singularly catastrophic health system. We bear the scars of a century of capitulation to those who value their profit over the health of our children. The basic knowledge of those institutions by which we are made healthy and safe has been made unnecessarily complicated. Failure to win this complicated game punishes you with meteoric destruction.

Against this, incrementalism can never work. Our goal is not a *slightly less bad* American health infrastructure. It is a *new* one, a *good* one—the best in the world. Within this abhorrent machine rests the potential to create a *singularly good* healthcare system. It is entirely within our power to wrest the basic human dignities of health and safety from those hands that hold the purse strings; it is within our collective ability to grant basic agency to all who wish to improve their conditions.

It is shameful to dream of anything less. It is a simple betrayal of the hungry, the poor, the immigrant, the disabled, the ailing—those people whose basic human dignity has been so thoroughly denied that it could never be satisfied by an army of small changes.

Pre-capitulating to the health insurance industry and its friends in the various half-measures presented above is an approach inadequate to the task of health justice. It is adequate only to the continual enrichment of private profit at the expense of those whom they have already harmed.

This is all a giant fraud perpetrated on the American people. We understand, as we have for decades, the interwoven problems of cost and coverage. We know, as we have always known, that the people who typically don't have insurance, or whose insurance is inadequate, are the people who are the most expensive to insure—and thus of the least interest to profit-seeking corporations. It has not been a surprise in my lifetime that rising costs are driven by rising prices, instead of irresponsible patients using healthcare resources "improperly." In real life, the fundamental myths upon which the insurance and healthcare industries insist reveal themselves to be smoke and deceit. But truth does not matter to the powerful. They hold our mediocre insurance plans hostage for government subsidy; a subsidy that lazy lawmakers would rather grant than interrogate the status quo of fear, profit, and domination in American healthcare.

But even if our state and if our corporations refuse to interrogate these structures, we can. The specter of healthcare spending haunts all these discussions: who spends it, who gets it, and what we try to do with it. Much of this spending is being aimed poorly. So let's talk about this money and how it's being spent—and the potential of single-payer to transcend these problems.

MONSTERS BIG AND SMALL

Taking care of a country requires spending quite a bit of money. This is obvious. It is also fine. Instead of finding ways to ax and slash our healthcare spending, to conceive narrowly of how it can be used and to hire an army of MBAs to optimize it, we should spend and invest our healthcare dollars wisely, for the betterment of all people.

I'm going to use a very dumb metaphor in this section. I'm going to talk about big monsters—think of dragons: colossal, devastating, and relentless; capable of leveling an entire city in one breath—and small monsters: goblins, or little imps; gnarly little perverts with daggers who attack in packs. I'm going to attempt to illustrate that we're spending our vast resources fighting off problems in American health finance that more resemble goblins when structural problems, like dragons— huge, powerful, catastrophic dragons—are already incinerating our communities.

In the past two decades goblins have been fashioned out of fears of "inefficient" or "low-value" care. We fear that some sinister or idiotic cohort of doctors is practicing medicine wastefully, and we fret that a simpleminded class of patients is seeking care recklessly. In this imagination, these individual doctors are the ones driving healthcare costs up for the rest of us. To combat this menace, insurers decided, we ought to simply *stop* providing "inefficient" care while continuing the normal course of "efficient" care—a procedure as simple as peeling a potato with a spoon. The presumption was that through the power of The Information Age™ we could seek out the goblins, precisely* excise the bad care from the good, and heroically bring prices down (without having to wonder why those prices were so high in the first place). This idea led us to the movement for "value-based payment."

"Quality" care and its "value-based" payment were fashioned as a national effort to subdivide the practice of medicine into an incomprehensible number of discrete pieces and measure them through long, bureaucratic processes designed by committees of committees. It develops payment schemes that are intended to reward "good" providers and punish "bad" ones. This idea has some merit: there are certainly providers who attempt to game the system; there are without question hospitals and healthcare corporations that abandon the public interest for their own profit. This payment system is meant

---

* Surgically, even!

well, and it's certainly not a unilaterally "bad" movement, but it is one inherently *distrustful* of doctors and patients, and it mistakes metrics for meaning.

The "quality" movement is focused on patient outcomes. But outcomes are driven just as much by the world in which patients exist outside the hospital—their housing, their food, their safety, their income—as by their medical condition before surgery. That's something that simply can't be and hasn't been measured well enough by this nitpicky obsession with "value." In the narrow way value-based payment sees it, hospitals with wealthier patients just tend to have better outcomes than hospitals with poorer ones. The complicated "quality" movement ultimately creates payment models in which hospitals that treat poorer patients are punished while hospitals that treat wealthier ones receive bonuses. We are trying to fight off our goblins but we're punishing people for having been caught in a dragon's path.

It manifests in other ways too. You, me, and every doctor and every patient, might intuit that these structural and social problems—our dragons—can be associated with, say, one's race and one's experience of structural racism. The consequences of structural racism saturate virtually every moment of a person's life, and therefore their health—but this urgent and obvious conclusion is unfathomable to the sterile "quality" measurement process. One could argue that quality-based payment models inadvertently discriminate against Black doctors, who disproportionately treat Black patients, for just this reason.[30]

But go deeper. Turn over the quality-obsessed ideology, like a mossy log in the woods, and underneath you'll find a nauseating, spongy, but firm belief in the permanence of the perverse forces that drive costs up. This is "just the way things are." If we believe there's just no way to halt rising costs, it follows that we must tighten our various belts and grit our assorted teeth and rub our few pennies together.

This is ridiculous: we are engaging in a titanic nickel-and-diming of doctors in order to cover for the innumerable massive healthcare corporations that are extorting us.

Only a federal universal single-payer has the ability to guarantee insurance for all people, the weight and force to reckon with the gross abuses in healthcare costs today, to lay waste to the goblin hordes, and the incentives and spending power to begin, after decades of neglect, to invest in the health of all tomorrow's patients.

And so the great task of a federal single-payer is to fight the *big* monsters, to vanquish dragons: to reckon with the corporate forces that seek to defraud us of hundreds of billions of dollars, and to spend generously on the care and the workers who provide it; which not only make us healthy *now*, but make us healthy in the future. But there is more to healthcare beyond the doctor's office or the hospital. And this is where the foulest monsters lurk.

★   ★   ★

Our highways are crumbling. Our trains, where they exist, are failing. Our sewer systems are disintegrating. So, too, is the health infrastructure of America. Under decades of for-profit domination, it has healed only some of us, while leaving the wounded rest behind. Over time, you and I are strung up for the vultures of capital to peck away at, and when nothing of us remains to interest them, we're discarded. Over time more and more of us wake up in the heap of left-behind bodies. Those of us who are yet cared for know we're just a snap of a thread we can't see from falling and being lost. Our neighborhoods have been made unsafe; our water has been made poisonous; we are hostages, trapped in our own bodies, to the billing departments of American healthcare.

Our money is wasted by the unworthy and uncaring, wasted on insurer advertising and administrative costs, and it can be won back only by switching to single-payer. There is money to be reclaimed by the weight and force of a single-payer's price-setting power. This is not "bonus" money; it is not money that can be given as appeasement or tribute to the wealthy and powerful; it is a small sliver of *our* money, which has for generations been stolen from us.

What do we do with *our* money?

We reclaim it, we invest it, and we rebuild. We use single-payer to liberate people from the torture of medical costs *and* reallocate our healthcare spending to take care of everyone in the long term.

We build primary care clinics in rural areas, where it's not profitable to stay open. We reopen the clinics—the 97 of them that have closed since 2010, plus unknown scores more in the decades before[31]—that tried to stave off the market's inevitable condemnation of caring for a sick but unprofitable rural population however they could,* until they collapsed.

We fund community health centers in poor neighborhoods; in communities that have been systematically preyed upon, drained of capital, punished for it, then punished again for suffering. These are communities that get sick more frequently, more severely, and in different ways than wealthier neighborhoods. This burden, compounded with each generation, will not be relieved by a program from a benevolent patrician class, but from a mass reversal of interwoven structural exploitations. A well-funded and well-staffed community health center, locally designed and locally controlled, can offer the specific kinds of care and support a community needs to stay

---

* In Copper Ridge, Tennessee, one rural hospital tried to raise the $100,000 required to stay open by crowdfunding on GoFundMe. They raised 3 percent of their goal.

healthy: direct healthcare and pharmacy services, social cooking classes, childcare and child development classes, and other vital resources to help a neighborhood stay healthy.[32]

Most importantly, we return the money to the people who do the work. We spoke earlier of the systemic underpayment of primary care providers, but there are millions of utterly devalued healthcare workers who through their labor are the backbone of American health: nurses, social workers,* custodial staff.

Take, for example, home-health aides like Kyle from the introduction to this book. It's one of the fastest-growing jobs in America: it's expected that there will be 1.2 million home-health aides by 2026.[33] Home-health services are billed at an average of $120 a visit, which is significantly cheaper than an inpatient stay at a hospital or nursing home.†

But gentle and convenient as this whole arrangement is, that money doesn't do much for the home-health aides themselves. For that $120 visit, these aides are paid a nationwide average of $11/hour—much, *much* lower in many states. The very same healthcare executives who found they could profit by denying patients home healthcare evolved to learn they could profit in the other direction by corporatizing it, contracting it out, and paying their workers as little as the local economy permits. They have folded and refolded the people who need long-term care and the people who provide it into crumpled, bloodied scrap.

The market won't solve this; the market *caused* this. So we use single-payer to allocate the money the private market has

---

* There are *so many* kinds of work that could be categorized as "social work," from the operator of the medical-legal partnership mentioned earlier to a translator in a hospital or immigrant health center.

† "The rates are fairly affordable with some home care agencies charging between $120 and $200 for every 10–12-hour overnight care." National Council for Aging Care, "In-home Care Costs Breakdown," https://aging.com/in-home-care-costs-breakdown/.

taken from us to do what it refuses: pay fair wages for essential care, which we guarantee to every person who needs it.

Is this not the most humane, the most just, the most *obvious* use of our collective wealth? Are we to believe that we should deprive ourselves from being a nation with well-paid home-health aides, or that we must keep their wages low so we can build another F-35?

I saw an excellent example of how investment in an expanded home-health labor force can produce better health outcomes when I visited a hospital in Little Rock, Arkansas. Arkansas, with high obesity and smoking rates, is one of the diabetes capitals of the United States. If you leave diabetes alone long enough, it'll erupt into a heart attack. So quite a few people from all around Pulaski County and beyond come to this hospital to seek treatment for cardiac failure. Often, they need pacemakers. But over a quarter of them are readmitted to the emergency department within a few weeks for cardiac complications or cardiac failure. That's not good. So this hospital, which was being penalized by Medicare for its high readmission rate, set out to bring these numbers down.*

Take a second to think about it. Who, or what, do you think most affects a person's chance of going back to the hospital after cardiac failure? Is it the quality or skill of their highly paid cardiologist? Is it the quality and engineering of their expensive pacemaker? Is it the $40,000 data package sold to hospi-

---

* This is an example of the odd assembly of "quality" measurements described previously. Certainly, it's not the hospital's "fault" that the people of Little Rock and beyond are more prone to cardiac failure than the people of, say, Sacramento, California, and are thus more likely to readmit to the hospital after heart failure. It might be, in fact, pretty unhelpful to penalize a hospital with sicker patients. But somebody needs to be made to care about bringing readmission rates down, and if the government refuses to invest in public well-being itself, the bureaucrats have to use various carrots and sticks (mostly sticks) to cajole private actors into doing it from their own profit interest.

tals* that lets nerds monitor pacemaker metrics? No, of course not—those are just the people who get to *bill* the most. What determines a person's likelihood of returning to the hospital are the living conditions and quality of life available to them. In this case: food and exercise.

So this hospital hired nurses, social workers, and nutritionists to see patients after their heart surgeries, to listen to them and ask them questions and encourage them to join Medicare-subsidized group classes at a hospital facility three times a week. There, patients join other patients of the same age group and heart condition to receive physical therapy, training, and exercise in a social environment. More importantly—for heart health is made, like abs, in the kitchen—they received group cooking classes, preparing (and eating) healthy food together.† The nurses proudly told me that readmission rates fell from 26 percent to 4 percent.

Our doctors, our diagnoses, our prescriptions, and our clinical time are often considered the fundamental components of healthcare. But that's shortsighted. We exist far beyond the walls of the hospital, and we are made healthy or ill long before a doctor sees us. Even after we see a doctor, our health outcomes are driven by non-diagnostic, extraclinical care: by social workers, by patient advocates, by nurses, by home-health workers, by the whole army of people who do the exhausting and tedious labor of being *nice* and *patient* with us. We are dependent upon their *compassionate labor.*‡ These are the people chronically unrecognized, underval-

---

* Sold to hospitals by corporations that share a major investor, nonetheless!

† The roadblocks to addressing obesity in America are many—primary among them, that many people can't afford and can't access healthy food, and don't have the time to prepare it if they can. This program addresses a different, but related issue: that the kind of diet that benefits cardiac health isn't necessarily the kind of comfort-food diet a 70-year-old Arkansan living outside Little Rock would have grown up with or chosen for him- or herself.

‡ What feminist writer Silvia Federici would describe as "feminized labor."

ued, and underpaid, and they're the primary actors who really make a difference in population health.

These are basic ideas! These are simple demands! We understand the social forces that make people healthy; we understand the structural forces that make people sick! Yet in the face of this knowledge that health has structural and social causes—knowledge we've had for decades—capitalism's response is to blame population illness on an aggregate of atomized individual choices, then package them into "healthy lifestyle" commodities. We're offered step trackers, cookbooks, various smartphone apps, all intended to somehow (it's not specified how) push or pull us into being "healthy"—at least long enough that we're no longer our insurance company's problem.

But despite what tech companies insist, there are no apps that bring about better health. A "how to survive on $4 a meal" cookbook, well-meaning as it may be,[34] doesn't do *shit* for people who only have $4, if that, per meal. Programs that penalize you for going to the ED at the wrong time don't do a single thing to make you healthier outside the hospital.

None of this is news. None of this is *new*. None of this would surprise a child. But somehow the multi-payer private model, in its half-century-long sandbox, has yet to figure this out. It hasn't even pretended to take it seriously. No private insurer has seriously invested in population health; none have invested in compassionate labor, or paying those laborers justly. And they never will.

Right now, your private insurer only bears the costs of you receiving care while they're insuring you. Because you're likely to change insurers in the future (sometimes every year), and eventually, god permitting, go on Medicare, they don't actually feel pressure to provide you with that which keeps you healthy, or that which helps you become healthier in the future. Solutions to the basic problems of health inequity elude private insurers not because they don't *understand* them; they understand them comprehensively; but because they refuse to reach—are *unable to* reach—for them. And their lazy poison drips from their slack jaws and infects the soil of American healthcare.

Let me put it another way.

You know that if your window is broken, the weather gets in. If the weather gets in, if you're exposed to the wind and snow of a Wisconsin winter or the suffocating wet heat of a Texas summer, you get sick. If you get sick, or if your kid gets sick, you have to go see a doctor.

But if there's no easy way to see a doctor—if the community clinic was shut down, or it's booked solid—you have to go to the hospital. If the hospital is far away, or if you don't have a car, you have to get a ride with a friend or neighbor, or you have to take the bus. In most parts of America, if you have to take the bus, you have to spend *all fucking day* dealing with the bus system.

If you have to spend all day dealing with the bus, you can't go to work.

And if you can't go to work, you can't afford to fix the window that caused the problem in the first place.

Your insurer, if you have one, will punish you for rushing to the hospital. You should've waited for an opening at the overbooked clinic, the bills they'll mail you will be meant to convey, or you should've called around to find an in-network family doctor. But how can you wait another day when your kid is sick? How can you endure when you had to get a coworker to cover your shift and you don't know if you can do it again?

The answer isn't to fork over a pile of cash every time you go to the hospital. The answer isn't to punish people for trying to get help. The answer begins with *giving people what they need* to fix the goddamn window.

But there are no private actors in the American model, no corporations or public-private partnerships, who will bear responsibility for fixing these problems on their own.

Consider the hookworm. Hookworm is a disease endemic to the deepest depths of poverty, one that we thought we had all but eradicated in the United States by the eighties.[35] We were wrong. Today, hookworm runs rampant through the poor and rural parts of the Deep South. The cause is devastating structural neglect. Sewer systems in rural counties—never intended to be stretched as thin as they are now—have fallen apart, or were constructed inadequately in the first place—and the state can't (or won't) approve the substantial funding required to retrofit them. So people make DIY fixes from PVC. These fixes break, and sewage piles up in people's yards.

In Lowndes County, Alabama—a rural county outside Montgomery, where a third of the population lives below the poverty line and nearly a quarter of people have diabetes—one in three people among a sample taken in 2017 had hookworm.[36] *One in three!* That's a rate consistent with (and, in many cases, higher than) devastated and impoverished countries.

In 2019, Blue Cross Blue Shield of Alabama has a monopoly on selling ACA insurance in Lowndes County.[37] They've had this monopoly for a few years now and, the way these things seem to work, will probably have a monopoly next year, too. Or maybe next year United will reenter the state for some reason and reclaim it, though I doubt it, because insurers tend only to enter new markets when those markets are urban areas with wealthy pockets. Either way, nothing will change.

The insurance industry is incapable of addressing the foundational problems of healthcare: of fixing the broken windows, of reopening the 16 rural hospitals that have closed in Texas because of lack of Medicaid funds since 2013,[38] of repairing the septic systems of Lowndes County—in almost the same way that a billionaire is incapable of lessening income inequality, or a cop is incapable of shrinking the prison-industrial complex. They cannot fix that injustice because they have been constructed by, and within, that injustice. They cannot solve these problems because they cannot exist without these problems, and thus existentially cannot *conceive* of them as problems in the first place.

But we can. And we do.

And so if private insurance companies are so shackled to their need for profit and are thus unable to feel the pain caused by their choices, if they do not suffer when those they insure suffer, and if they continue to make choices that cause more and more pain to others, and are by their very nature unable to keep themselves from doing so, then we simply should replace them.

It makes perfect sense that the actor that *does* suffer when its people *don't* get care—all of us, united against suffering, our bodies together assembled in the shape of our government—should be the actor that also *guarantees* that care in the first place.

This is the transformative potential of single-payer.

PART III:

WHAT LIES BEYOND

Once the federal actor—the single payer—bears the costs of providing our care and the risks and costs of what happens when care is *not* provided, once we force it to confront the suffering of all its people, it can finally be used as a tool for realizing *health justice*. It becomes the only extension of our democratic government that feels, and that can be made accountable for, the strain of America's collective miseries. It is forced, in a way that no other government program is forced, to reckon with the financial consequences of health inequity—and that might have the power and resources to address them.

We witness the final marks of health inequity in the clinic, the hospital, the graveyard. But they are branded upon us much earlier—in the neighborhood, in the home, in the womb. If we wish to address health inequity, to heal the wounds of health injustice, our goal becomes to not just treat the illness, but to resolve or prevent that which makes us ill.

In this final part of the book, I will discuss some of the causes of health inequity and their structural roots. This section is not meant to serve as a zoo of suffering people. It would be insufficient to simply catalog the flavors of American agony. Rather, I reckon that we have been atomized in our suffering. We have been persuaded that the ways we hurt are fundamentally disjointed from one another, and we are encouraged to submit to this alienation from the people around us.

I reject this notion. Our tears all fall into the same deep basin. Health inequity—health injustice—is written, long or short, upon each of us in the same hand. I hope to illustrate the depth and breadth of how it manifests, in both the structural and personal; and then, at the end, I'll explain why I believe this means there is a shared cause in our different struggles to help ourselves and the people we love.

THE SOCIAL DETERMINANTS OF HEALTH

Health policy has a term I like: the "social determinants of health." They are just what they say on the box: the social and societal factors that determine your health status. Remember from earlier in the book that access to healthcare (varied as it is) only represents a fifth of the known difference between different people's health outcomes? These determinants make up much, if not all, of the rest.[1]

Social determinants are the constellation of extraclinical factors—things that happen outside the hospital or doctor's office—that shape how, why, and how severely a person becomes ill. In many cases, they're more influential than the quality of treatment in patient outcomes. Whether or not a person will recover after surgery is, in large part, determined long before they are admitted to the hospital. If you want to reduce maternal mortality, for example, but you only intervene at the time of delivery, you're too late.

Just as a person with no place to live or no food to eat is likely to face worse health outcomes and require more (and more expensive) healthcare than a person with a safe home and a healthy diet, people who have been denied other social determinants will be sicker, die sooner, and require more medical care (which, under the current American model, they are unlikely to be able to access). They are as much "healthcare" as is penicillin or a knee replacement.

Unlike illnesses, social determinants are (as the name implies) social constructs. The body is that strange bag of unknowable goo, and no law on Earth can govern the movements of blood or tissue. Whether a person gets asthma, lupus, borderline personality disorder, or cancer is in large part uncontrollable and irreversible (even if the disorder can be treated). But the social conditions that make those illnesses more likely or more severe are absolutely within our control. There is no law of nature that denies every person in America a safe place to sleep or healthy food to eat. There is only an institutional refusal to see it provisioned.

Here are some of these social determinants and their role in American health.

HOUSING

If your people are suffering because they don't have a place to live, or if the places they live are unsafe, then **housing is healthcare**, and you must build safe social housing to reduce healthcare inequity and bring healthcare costs down.

Exposure to a Chicago winter or a Phoenix summer kills faster than cancer. People who are chronically homeless are at higher risk of many kinds of severe illnesses (including cancer), report a rate of mental illness several times higher than that of housed people, and have a life expectancy about 25 years shorter than the rest of the population.[2] And by virtue of their homelessness—not a personal or moral failing, but representative of a national refusal to recognize a right to shelter or let people have a place to live—they are also very expensive to take care of.

This is all intuitive and hardly radical. Every emergency nurse in every hospital in America knows the list of "frequent utilizer" patients who show up over and over and over again either because they don't have a home and don't have any other place to go in extreme weather, or because they have a serious medical problem and nowhere to live and nowhere to receive regular care.* These conditions make them very expensive to treat, and they need care frequently. As institutions with money begin to feel the pressure of these hospital admissions, they've gradually decided to experiment with investing in housing.

New York's Medicaid program has spent hundreds of millions of dollars on its Supportive Housing Initiative, targeted at Medicaid recipients who are particularly expensive (similar to the general cost curve in American healthcare, a fifth of the state's Medicaid recipients have significant medical needs and require three-quarters of its Medicaid dollars).[3] This program, which includes things like subsidized rent, housing assistance, and budgeting for direct housing construction, reduces the time each patient spends in the hospital by 60 percent after a year of housing, and lessens their overall Medicaid spending by about $6,000 per person.[4] In Chicago, the University of Illinois hospital started a program to provide a small number of unhoused patients (whose frequent hospital visits cost the hospital an average of $1,500 a night) with government-subsidized housing and a social worker to help them transition and manage their long-term health needs. They saw a reduction in per-patient costs of 18 percent and, after the pilot, doubled the size of the program.[5] In Portland, Oregon, and Orlando, Florida, hospitals are directly funding the construction of housing, citing similar arguments about reducing hospital use and cost.

What's unsaid in these stories is that the only reason hospitals are investing in housing is that they're compelled by federal legislation to stabilize anyone who enters their emergency department: they have been inadvertently forced to bear some long-term costs of homelessness. Is this the patchwork model by which we want to understand housing as healthcare? Must we determine someone's worthiness of a home by whether

---

* This is a problem of similar shape to the revolving door of homeless people and people with mental health issues in prisons.

their individual homelessness costs a particular company too much money? Despite the best intentions of hospitals like U of I, they're housing people a couple dozen at a time—while there are thousands of people still sleeping outside, well beyond the capability of any hospital to treat.

It is not only the absence of housing that affects healthcare. We are made sick by the quality and safety of our housing. We fall sick if those homes are polluted or full of mold. Unsafe homes punish children with lifelong developmental and respiratory illnesses for the sin of being born poor, for growing up drinking poison and breathing spores. Sometimes the only housing available to poor people is cramped, poorly constructed or maintained, tumbledown structures—and sometimes these homes are death traps. Despite its location in one of the wealthiest boroughs of London, the dilapidated Grenfell Tower fire's death toll of 74 counted only poor among its rank. There was no affordable safe housing for those people who were lost in Oakland's Ghost Ship. Immolation is a death reserved for the poor.

FOOD

If your people are suffering because they don't have access to healthy food to eat, or they don't have any food at all—and so they're getting diabetes or comorbidities of diabetes like cardiac failure—then **food is healthcare**, and you must provide them with affordable or free food options, as well as the time, space, and materials required to prepare them. This will reduce health inequity and bring healthcare costs down.

In America, food-related health problems come in two varieties: those of not having enough food, also known as food insecurity, and those of not eating (or having access to) the right kinds of food.

About 50 million Americans faced food insecurity in 2013.[6] Of the food-insecure families served by food bank network Feeding America in 2014, over half were forced to choose between food and utilities, transportation, medical care, or rent. In other words: nearly a tenth of American families have to choose between their meals and their medicine, or their meals and their housing. Food insecurity correlates with serious health conditions that can linger for an entire life: worsened nutritional and mental health in youth,[7] diabetes and hypertension in adults,[8] and significant physical impairment to senior citizens. (Per one study, "seniors experiencing food insecurity are more likely to have limitations in activities of daily living akin to a food-secure senior 14 years older.")[9]

The other food problem is diet. In many parts of the country, urban and rural, it's relatively easy to access calorie-rich, convenient, and inexpensive unhealthy food, and relatively difficult to obtain or prepare healthier food. When people eat unhealthily over a sustained period of time they run the risk of becoming obese or getting diabetes, conditions that significantly affect their long-term health outcomes and risk of medical complications.[10] You've probably heard the term "food desert," a term that describes an area without access to affordable healthy food. This is, of course, an entirely man-made phenomenon in which the free market decides it just isn't *profitable* to sell affordable healthy food to people in poor neighborhoods.

Unlike the example of housing, there is no single actor who bears the costs for society's long-term problems of food— perhaps Medicaid comes closest, if anyone. Hunger is sated quickly, but nutrition's effects on the body take time to develop; solutions to food problems might take a decade to be fully digested. As a result, there are fewer flashy high-dollar public-private partnerships to tout, and those that do exist focus primarily on diet. In 2010, the Obama administration carried forth the banner of public-private partnerships and approved the Healthy Food Financing Initiative, which spent $220 million to incentivize supermarkets to move into food deserts, mostly through subsidies. While it helped grocery stores open in underserved areas, it could not guarantee people could afford the resulting accessible food and failed to change diets among the people it targeted.[11]

Which makes sense, right? Like housing, food access does not seem to be a thing that can be solved by properly incentivizing for-profit entities to take care of it. The food desert is an abstraction of the problems driven by our collective failure to ensure all people have the food they need and just placing grocery stores in a neighborhood does not necessarily fix any of these problems. Healthy food is more expensive than unhealthy food, and people without a lot of money are less likely to buy it, even if the store selling it is within walking distance. Supermarkets in poor neighborhoods are less likely to sell healthy food than supermarkets in richer ones.[12]

"Access" alone is insufficient. Just as "access to healthcare" or, even worse, "affordable access," does nothing for the person with expensive health problems, "food access" is inadequate to solve the problems of being unable to afford food, or lacking time to prepare it. "Access" alone paves the way for the goblins of "personal responsibility," which let policy-makers write off suffering as being a natural consequence of the sufferer's choices; that diabetes could have been avoided if only the poor patient had pinched their pennies and bought more kale. How degrading a worldview.*

---

*   It is worth noting that much of our wildly unhealthy food is the product of a farm subsidy system that prioritizes the destructive overproduction of corn, and a century of food science that turns it, alchemy-like, into addictive and incredibly unhealthy food products that can be sold much more cheaply than healthier options. In this sense, the American diabetes epidemic is an end-to-end capitalist affliction: https://www.nationalgeographic.com/people -and-culture/food/the-plate/2016/07/are-corn-subsidies-making-us-fat-/.

A proper solution to food and health inequity cannot be summoned up from the dregs of public-private partnerdom, but a good start might look like the community health center in Detroit, which offers cooking classes to its neighbors, or Medicare- or Medicaid-sponsored meal delivery services for elderly or disabled people.

By bearing responsibility for paying for the long-term costs of food inequity, after they manifest in the hospital, a single-payer program can be forced to feel the agony of starvation of malnutrition in a way private insurance can't and won't, and it can support the relatively simple and cheap programs that might alleviate it: kitchens, robust and generous food pantries, and community spaces for cooking and eating.

MORE SOCIAL DETERMINANTS OF HEALTH

The problems of housing and food are not big-brain nerd problems like "How do we go to Mars?" They are problems with easy-to-understand solutions and resources readily available in America. As it stands, though, nobody feels the pressure and heat to act; to sponsor the simple solutions to suffering. But by virtue of the relationship between the social determinants of health and health costs, we can use single-payer to build pressure to demand this accountability from the state.

Our government, and the people who run it, are happy to reap the rewards of our collective labor and our collective triumphs.* But this relationship only runs one way: our government has self-insulated, and refuses to suffer when its people suffer. This is a wonderful piece of magicianship, because the state has made sure that the consequences of the problems it permits—lack of housing, lack of food, a broken healthcare

---

*   It then, of course, redistributes these rewards to those who are already wealthy.

system—will not afflict the state directly or fiscally. The state can "feel" only through its finances; when a child goes hungry or a homeless person freezes to death or a family receives a $40,000 bill for an emergency room visit, the state spends nothing and feels nothing. Austerity and "fiscal responsibility" are the tools for the American state to deny accountability for the American suffering it has permitted, or even caused, all in the service of its total capitulation to the interests of people who have money and power.

And so the goal is to force ourselves to suffer collectively when one among us suffers—to pay gladly the full sum of our healthcare costs—and to use our great assembled might to work to ensure that nobody need suffer again.

If your people are suffering because their ground has been made toxic, if their water has been made poisonous, if the places they live have been made lethal, then **environmentalism is healthcare**, and you must provide the rehabilitation, relocation, and resuscitation of both person and earth to bring healthcare costs down. The people of Flint, Michigan, have been poisoned with lead after crumbling city infrastructure exposed water mains to corrosion. Lead poisoning can take decades to reveal itself, and Flint's children will likely suffer lifelong cognitive and neurological impairment.[13] Milwaukee, too, faces a similar crisis: gentrification construction jostled water pipes in poor and Black neighborhoods, knocking lead into the water—a crisis to which the city has been humiliatingly inadequate in its response.[14] In San Francisco, the Bayview–Hunters Point neighborhood has seen a decades-long cover-up of the toxic waste that's been dumped and ignored in the backyards of poor families, people of color, and public housing. It was hardly a secret—the people who live there know what's up. They know why their life expectancy is 14 years shorter than the life expectancy in Nob Hill, just three miles north. But nobody listened to them. After a 15-year city cover-up—

eventually revealed by a determined local reporter—the desecration of Bayview–Hunters Point only registered among the
wealthier types because YIMBY* dipshits and their waxy-faced
wieners in city hall want to use the neighborhood to throw up
more condos for rich goobers.†

If your schools are in shambles, falling apart around their students; if your teachers don't have the supplies, space, or training
to teach; if the classroom holds nothing for its children and, in
turn, its children abandon it—then you must understand that
education is healthcare. Educational attainment very strongly
correlates with health outcomes, both direct mortality and the
adoption of important health behaviors.[15] Both are true: health
is a prerequisite to education, and education also improves
health. Children with more access to educational opportunities
(holding constant other factors like income and school quality)
smoke less, drink less, and have fewer health conditions two
decades later. This effect, like many, compounds across generations. Babies born to pregnant people with less education are
more likely to die before their first birthday.[16] One study found
each additional year of education associates with a 7–9 percent
decline in infant mortality.[17]‡

---

* YIMBY stands for "Yes in My Backyard," a reference to (usually racist) "Not in
  My Backyard" antidevelopment activists. They are generally yuppie dipshits
  who believe the housing market can solve our problems of housing, if only
  we let developers *build*. That they will only build expensive condos is not
  factored into this equation. Perhaps the condos will "trickle down" to poor
  or working-class people who are priced out of the neighborhood.

† It's worth noting that the Pelosi and Feinstein families have invested in the
  construction and development projects in Bayview–Hunters Point.

‡ I wouldn't advocate for educational equity exclusively because of health
  outcomes in pregnancies. Educational attainment should be celebrated in
  its own right, and it's already too often that our society values a woman or
  pregnant person on whether or not they have a kid. However, the results
  are striking and expose the strong linkage between important educational
  programs, like universal pre-K and free college for all, and health equity.

To a large degree, both intra- and intergenerational effects are tied to a web of underlying factors like income, neighborhood safety, and parental involvement. A family with the resources to afford a healthy pregnancy and delivery, plus active participation in a child's education, is more likely to show better long-term health outcomes. When families are provided safe and competent education, and (like food) have the time and space to use it, they benefit: in one study, children from poor families in Chicago who were given educational enrichment from pre-kindergarten to third grade showed "lower rates of out-of-home placement (indicating child abuse), lower rates of arrests and conviction for violent behaviors, and lower rates of disability" compared to children from similar neighborhoods by age 24.[18] This fight, too, is one of healthcare.

If your people can't afford the necessities of life—food, shelter, medicine—or if affording a basic existence comes at such a cost that they're left ragged and hurting, then you understand that **income is healthcare**. Poverty haunts us from cradle to grave: lower income is associated with higher infant mortality and shorter lifespans.[19] If, in 2014, all states had increased their minimum wage by one dollar, there would have been 2,790 fewer low-birth-weight births and 518 fewer postneonatal deaths.[20] There exists a hideous strain of wretched thought that posits that suffering associated with impoverishment stems from a "culture of poverty," or some innate crudeness among the lower classes, whose ignorance and foul dirtiness cause their own ruin. This is loathsome and lazy thinking. The problems associated with poverty are not caused by "culture." They are caused by *poverty* and the thousand hateful barnacles that cling to and depend upon it: the double jeopardies of impoverishment and structural racism; of impoverishment and dysfunctional, underfunded schools; of impoverishment and lack of medical facilities. This happens both to people and to places. Where the slow rampage of capitalism has poisoned the land, closed the factories, and left behind only abandoned buildings—where there are no jobs to be had, and nobody can make a promise of a better tomorrow—health outcomes plummet. Deindustrialization, for example, is understood to be a risk factor for opioid addiction.[21] And so if you care, or if you have been compelled to care, about the health of your people, you must invest in the slow work of liberating all people from poverty; of tilting against the centuries of exploitation and immiseration for profit.

We are woven to one another and our surroundings; we are wrapped in fractal webs of gossamer thread that bind us to those forces, seen and unseen, that determine how we live and how we die. And if all these things are healthcare, and if all these things dictate our health outcomes and drive our healthcare costs, and if all these things are, more often than not, imposed upon us, and if we have the ability—and we do—to ameliorate the misery they inflict upon our neighbors and communities, don't we have the obligation, by our simple moral constitution, to do it? Don't we have the resources, through single-payer financing, to realize and benefit from it?

HOUSTON JAILS AS WAREHOUSES FOR THE SICK

Let me describe how single-payer is woven into a broader tapestry of health justice by talking about Houston, Texas, jail, and mental health.

I moved to Houston as a teenager for college and consider it as much my hometown as central Wisconsin, where I grew up. It's a sprawling concrete swamp with heinous summers, and it is (despite the bus system's best efforts) challenging to navigate without a car; it's a place with a long and continuing history of violent structural racism; and it's also home to several million generally warm and unpretentious people, my favorite rap music, and scenes of great and bizarre beauty, both natural and unnatural (plus arguably the greatest variety of cheap and delicious food of any major American city). I visit several times a year, sometimes to give talks about healthcare to any audience willing to listen.

But you can't talk about healthcare without talking about mental health. (Or, rather, you *shouldn't*. Clearly America's insurance companies—who understand mental health services to be long-term profit-drainers—are very good at drawing lines between "health" and "mental health.") And you can't talk about mental health in Houston without talking about Harris County Jail, the largest "provider" of mental health resources in the city and, by extension, in all of Texas.[22]

I have this same conversation with different nouns across the whole goddamn country. You talk about mental healthcare in Austin, and Travis County Jail comes up. In New York, it's Rikers Island. Wisconsin—Milwaukee County Jail. Hell, in Chicago you speak to anyone about healthcare, and it's not long before someone mentions that Cook County Jail is the largest provider of mental health services in not just Chicago, but the entire country.[23]

That's a necessary and functional observation, but it doesn't really explain adequately the mechanism by which the delegation of mental health services to the carceral state happens, or what it looks like. So let's talk about that.

I had the chance to speak with Franklin Bynum, a former public defender and socialist who, in 2018, was elected a judge in Harris County's criminal circuit as part of a massive wave of reform candidates, including a coalition of 17 Black women who challenged Republican incumbents. While a public defender, Bynum worked with people who were suspected of having a mental illness. He walked me through the judicial process by which the link between mental health and prison is forged.

Every morning that he served as public defender, Bynum woke up to a list of names of people who had been arrested recently and were believed to have mental health disorders. They were held in the Harris County Courthouse, a sleek and pretty modern building in downtown Houston, where, if you looked out from a window just a few stories up, you could see both a bail bond lender and a former slave market.[*] Detainees are held behind each courtroom in dark, dank, dungeonesque cells, so thoroughly hidden from public view that if you were to visit the courthouse, you might never know these holding cells exist.

Bynum would enter a cell and introduce himself to the detainee. If the detainee were capable of introducing themself and understanding who Bynum was and what his job was, then, in order to help the detainee, Bynum had to help them plead guilty. Not because the detainee was necessarily guilty—but because judges typically refuse to release people on personal bond, and set cash bond far, far out of the reach of the common defendant.

If you're a person with a mental illness who has already been locked up for several days without the medication you need to function—in all likelihood, for nonviolent offenses like trespassing or disorderly conduct—the coercion of this arrangement is overwhelming. Plead guilty, and you might get out on time served. Fight it, and you're looking at more time locked up without care. So people plead guilty to things they shouldn't have to just so they can get their medicine.

This also has the side effect of "speeding the docket" for the courthouse so the judge looks more productive and has less work to do.

Frankly, this grim scenario presumes the detainee is *lucky*

---

[*]   If this were a literary construction, it might be edited out for being too "on the nose."

enough to pass as functioning normally. If the detainee is unable
to identify themself, if they're in the middle of a serious mental health episode, if they were to declare to Bynum that they
were the "king of Houston" or otherwise indicate a paranoid
or hallucinatory episode, things become more drastic. Now the
detainee is held longer—up to 30 days—until the county can
provide a brief session with a psychiatrist. The detainee is held
in a hospital wing of the prison, or a prison wing of a hospital.

There's this concept of the "prison-to-hospital" pipeline that
comes up when talking about people with mental illnesses in
jail. Except pipelines are generally orderly and unidirectional.
Here, it's more like a pinball machine. Giant, invisible flippers
bounce people around, from jail to hospital to jail to hospital,
and at some point, there's no functional difference between
the two. We refuse to care for people, and so they become sick.
We make them sick. And if you're the wrong kind of sick, or if
you're the wrong kind of person, we delegate your care to the
prisons, which are becoming increasingly privatized.

I mean, hell, you can't look at the opioid epidemic in
America without witnessing our massive and almost entirely
carceral response to it—a call from a playbook tested mostly
on Black and Brown people during the War on Drugs. There's a
whole generation of children out there who barely know their
parents because we decided their parents' sickness is a crime,
and one for which the only solution is lockup, not treatment (a
standard, of course, never set for people who have money), and
never, under any circumstances, actual *relief.*

It's technically not a crime to be poor, it's technically not
a crime to be sick, it's technically not a crime to be Black
or Brown, but once you fall into the intersections, the rules
change on you. If you're a poor single mother of color, for
example—you have virtually no right to privacy.[24] If you're
in Section 8 housing, a state agent comes to your apartment
twice a month and counts the shoes on your shoe rack. If they

find too many, or if you're a single mother and they find a *man's* shoes, you can lose your benefits.* If you're disabled and on Medicaid, every month a nurse comes to your house to check if you're still disabled, or if you're faking it. If you're a Medicaid recipient in a work requirements state, every month you gotta wait in line for hours at an intentionally understaffed office to prove that you're employed. These are frustrating, confusing forces, sculpted by human hands, that drive people into jails. So long as we use prison to hide those who have been made "undesirable," healthcare and prison are inseparable.

While it is well-intentioned and technically correct to claim that prisons are the largest providers of mental healthcare in the United States, the technicalities mask great suffering. Prisons might dispense what are legally categorized as "mental health services," but (as the brilliant prison abolitionist Mariame Kaba points out) they don't provide mental health*care*.[25] So long as they are behind bars, no prisoner will receive the care, support, or resources they need to handle whatever illness has damned them to incarceration in the first place; no prisoner will be saved from the inevitable reincarcerations when that illness persists beyond the bars.

Prisons are not hospitals. They are *warehouses for the mentally ill*. They are storage units for the unwanted.

The Democrats, the liberals, they know this is bad. And luckily, they have a plan. A few years ago I volunteered on a project for the Laura and James Arnold Foundation (LJAF), also based in Houston.† The LJAF is a huge do-gooder foundation funded by some portion of the billions of dollars John Arnold made in energy trading. It seeks, generally, to fund

---

*   This has a haunting and more explicit predecessor in the welfare restrictions of the seventies and eighties. Until *King v. Smith* in 1968, a single mother's welfare could be denied if caseworkers found that she was *having sex with men*. For more evidence of patriarchal domination rampant in welfare "means-testing," see https://www.motherjones.com/politics/2009/01brave-new-welfare/.

†   It was not explained to us how our work would be used.

so-called "data-driven" reforms. They wanted to understand what predicts recidivism—that is, why do people who go to jail go back to jail? So they took these three brilliant data scientists, plus me, and we got our little *Mission: Impossible*–cleanroom–style virtual machine, and we looked at police records and jail data and courthouse records. After all this hemming and hawing, after all this brainpower and technical expertise, we discovered that the people who go to jail most often, and who return to jail after going to jail, are people who are arrested for the crime of being homeless. They get arrested for being homeless, they go to jail for being homeless, then they get released and remain homeless.

This is a *revelation* for these people.

The LJAF takes projects like these and, at least in Houston, is building little opaque computers for judges that indicate whether it thinks a given defendant should receive the less cumbersome personal recognizance bond, or an impossible cash bond. The computer—a kind of black box—aggregates historical data on people who have previously been sentenced to jail to determine who should be given basic empathy. Since the history of incarceration has disproportionately affected poor people, people of color, and sick people,* the black box also disproportionately suggests that these people continue being detained under bonds they can't afford—in precisely the same way as they were before. Not much has changed—except this time, a computer tells the judge they're doing the right thing.

The Arnold Foundation understands that cash bail unnecessarily harms people. In fact, they're very concerned about it.

---

* The LJAF argues that their black boxes are "race blind" because their data sets exclude fields like race. It doesn't take very long to realize that a data set of *people who are arrested in Houston* is going to overrepresent people of color, sick people, and poor people. The quality of their algorithm is unknowable, as they consider it proprietary and refuse to submit it to public review, even as they push for its placement in courtrooms.

It's just that their vision of a better world is one in which some people are *necessarily harmed*, and we have a chart to tell us that they deserve it.

This is the neoliberal approach to the carceral state. Not to dismantle it, but to rationalize it. To invent processes that reenact already-existing acts of structural violence—the dehumanization of poor, sick, and Black or Brown people—then cite those old acts of violence as justification for the new acts of violence. It is a tautological model of immiseration.

HEALTH JUSTICE

Here is why I opened the third act of a book about single-payer—and why I introduced its first real discussion of mental health—by talking about Houston jails. Mental health is obviously a matter of healthcare, and one that the federal single payer can comfortably offer immediate short-term assistance but limited long-term solutions for. A single payer can pay for mental healthcare and medications without passing costs to the patients. It can lower the price of medication with size and negotiating power.* Maybe it can even lead to the public pro-

---

*   This is a limited solution. One flaw in the idea that a single-payer can simply "negotiate prices down" for all drugs is that negotiation presumes the payer is willing to walk away, or has other options it can use. This is true in the case of, say, antibiotics, or other drugs with multiple competitors or generic options—the single-payer can refuse to play ball and go with a cheaper option. But this is not effective for expensive drugs with no market competition or that treat relatively few patients. Consider, for example, the hepatitis C drug making budgeting difficult for many states with high rates of Opioid Use Disorder (OUD). In theory, the federal payer can afford to pay pharma's prices, but that's virtually indistinguishable from ransom. Instead, I'm interested in something else. Especially considering that so much foundational pharmaceutical research is done by under or unpaid grad students in American universities, doesn't it make sense for America to reimagine pharmaceuticals as utility, and take on public production for public benefit?

duction of drugs. It can even attempt to address our current provider shortage (the fact that there simply aren't enough psychologists and psychiatrists) by increasing payment for patient care.

What single-payer cannot do of its own accord is solve problems beyond the clinic or heal the underlying wounds that inflict these miseries in the first place. It is entirely possible to imagine a world in which single-payer is real and people with mental health needs are still jammed into jail cells; a world in which we all visit a doctor whenever we need it without receiving a bill but people whose primary crime is being sick are still warehoused in the prison. When single-payer is passed, and I believe it will be passed, the people we love will still be homeless, will still be poor, will still live on poisoned land, will still be compelled into sickness. If our solutions to human misery are like those of the foundations and the think-tankers and the reasonable policy people—if they are rooted in the implicit justification of some portion of that misery—we will never achieve relief.

If we believe in the promise of single-payer to help us demand accountability for the structural problems that plague us, we cannot imagine it as a satisfactory endpoint. We cannot fight for health justice without fighting those forces that make people unwell in the first place.

Health policy is the power of life and death. We must demand nothing less than its public control. To set our aims anywhere else is to be satisfied with insurance. Essential, tremendous, life-changing universal comprehensive insurance—but, still, insurance.

Insurance is not enough. Our goal is not just insurance, but emancipation. We must put the people who have been most harmed at the front of the line. We must walk together every step of the way. We must never compromise until all of us have been liberated.

THE STRUCTURAL DETERMINANTS OF HEALTH

Liberated how? From what?

The framework of health justice emphasizes that the material things that affect our daily lives also affect our health. Medicine is complicated, but the basic structure of public health needn't be: if you are deprived of the things you need to stay healthy, it follows that you'll become sick. So why do some people have these social determinants, and others don't? Why do some people have housing, food, and income, while others are left in the dirt?

Why and how these social determinants appear isn't random. There are causes, underlying forces that dictate their arc of deprivation and misery and their impacts on health. I'm going to call these underlying forces the *structural determinants of health*. Let's talk about what I see as the big three: racism, sexism, and poverty.

RACISM

In America, people of color are more likely than white people to report being in poor health. For a given health condition, Black people are more likely than white people to suffer worse outcomes.[*] As a result, there's a widely held conclusion, even among the academics and other nerdlinger-types in health policy, that health outcomes differ by race. This conclusion is lazy. Health outcomes don't differ because of *race*. They differ because of *racism*.

---

[*]   Hispanic people tend to have outcomes better than Black people, but this obfuscates a wide variety of differences among different ethnic groups that make up the Hispanic label. Puerto Ricans are 1.2 to 1.5 times more likely to suffer from cancer and heart disease than Mexican Americans, for example.

There is no racial propensity for infant death that explains why Black infants die at more than twice the rate—11.4 per thousand—of white infants.[26] There is no innate characteristic of Black men that predisposes them to live five years shorter than white men.[27] (Not for lack of searching: in 2007, Oprah and Dr. Oz posited a theory that those slaves who had survived the brutal, grotesque Middle Passage were more able to retain salt than those slaves who died, thus passing on a genetic predisposition for salt retention, leading to higher rates of fatal hypertension. This theory was convincingly debunked 15 years before it appeared on TV.)[28] Instead, it is the brutal and numerous minglings of structural racism and its effects that are etched into the bodies of people of color in America.

The ways in which this happens run a spectrum as broad and varied as the American creativity for reimagining white supremacy. Immigrants, for example, whose jobs often don't come with insurance, find themselves with restricted access to healthcare, or put off seeking urgent care out of fear of deportation or punishment. This is not alleviated by citizenship; in fact, perversely, it often gets worse—children of immigrants, and children of children of immigrants, have more health conditions (like developmental problems, learning disabilities, or respiratory illness) and worse health outcomes than their parents.[29] There's a selection effect here—the United States's rigid immigration policies make it more difficult for sick people to immigrate—but the generational worsening of immigrant health is soundly demonstrated and yet difficult to examine. Racial minorities in America face not only difficulty accessing good care, but receive worse care when they can get it. They also encounter more actively harmful health factors, like unsafe or polluted neighborhoods—even more so if they're poor. To many immigrants, especially ethnic minorities, America simply makes you sick.[30]

Urban segregation is a readily visible and physically tangible consequence of structural racism with an obvious impact on health. In 2001, at least six major American cities were about as segregated as South Africa was during apartheid.* Black and Hispanic neighborhoods in segregated cities have more concentrated poverty, poorer public schools, worse and more cramped housing, and a higher rate of regular exposure to environmental hazards.[31] This has not happened by accident—it is the result of decades and decades of racially motivated choices by city councils, mortgage brokers, urban planners, and federal lenders. These social determinants of health were assigned by racist malice.

All of this is *stressful*. That stress—the repetitive onslaught of social, psychological, physical, and chemical stressors, racism both actively and passively experienced, packed and hardened over time—has health consequences. Everyday discrimination has been linked to a host of negative health outcomes, from coronary artery calcification[32] to high blood pressure[33] to lower birth weight.[34]

This is not simply reducible to wealth or "socioeconomic status"; racism is intermingled with, but distinct from, economic exploitation. When income, condition severity, and other factors are controlled, Black men with cardiac conditions receive less diagnostic care than white men while receiving invasive procedures more frequently.[35]

Atop this foundation, there are built racialized differences in American responses to health crises. We generally understand that the opioid epidemic in America is driven more by illness than a crime wave. Some states and cities debate or

---

* This is determined using a "dissimilarity index," which measures "the percentage of a group that would have to move in order for that group to be evenly distributed across a metropolitan area." See "Race, Racial Inequality and Health Inequities: Separating Myth from Fact," edited by Brian Smedley, Michael Jeffries, Larry Adelman and Jean Cheng.

even roll out sweeping, comprehensive programs to treat opioid use disorder like an addiction instead of an epidemic of
criminal mentality. This is obviously the moral and correct
way to handle Opioid Use Disorder (OUD): with rehab, with
therapy, with pain management, with decriminalization, and
with empathy. But this was not the case during the crack epidemic, which carried with it horror stories of urban warfare
and gang affiliations and a new, unstoppable breed of Black
child "superpredators"—a heinously racist myth endorsed by
a sitting U.S. president!

The American response to the old epidemic of addiction
was aggressively carceral, to the point that we disappeared
an entire generation of Black men. The American response to
the new one features wall-to-wall command centers, national
debates, the language of safety and reintegration.* Cops bring
NARCAN to middle-class white neighborhoods with high
numbers of OUD calls. They bring guns to Black and Brown
and poor ones.

SEXISM

Heavy is the hammer that beats down upon women and trans
people. One statistic is so raw and so heinous that it's broken
through into pop culture: America's maternal mortality rate
is the highest in the so-called "first world." Twenty-six mothers die for every 100,000 live births.[36] That's almost three times
higher than in the UK, and nearly seven times higher than in
Finland.[37]

If most premature deaths are avoidable, and they are, it's
these deaths during and after delivery that are most flagrant in

---

* It is also deeply carceral and punitive, especially for poor people, but it at least
  has components of something more compassionate.

their absurd cruelty. Half of these deaths could have been prevented—not through lifestyle changes or long-term courses of medication, but through simple, common clinical procedures.[38] Doctors habitually ignore or underestimate mothers' reports of pain, especially when those patients are Black mothers, and then are surprised when that pain stems from complications that require urgent care. Mothers bleed out on the operating table because their physicians and nurses don't take their blood pressure at appropriate intervals. Amniotic fluid or postoperative wounds become infected after delivery and aren't caught or treated in time.

Here, as elsewhere, there is not a uniform distribution of misery. Black mothers die during childbirth at over three times the rate of white mothers.[39] This is a pain not prevented by individual wealth or power: even Serena Williams, the greatest professional athlete of our generation, found her symptoms ignored by her medical staff, and came close to death during her own delivery.[40]

Then there are those who are powerless and pregnant. So-called "fetal protection laws," passed by a set of reactionary legislators in over a dozen states, conjure up myths of "crack babies" and their resulting costs to the welfare state, to target pregnant people* who are battling drug addiction. These pregnant people are disproportionately poor people and people of color. Someone who presents signs of drug usage at a prenatal visit, or who tests positive for crack, can be shackled and thrown in jail—again, the warehouse for the undesired—where they will give birth on a metal slab, arms and legs bound.[41]

Shackled delivery is made yet more disgusting by the fact that fetal exposure to crack, in isolation, has not been linked to any discovered disorder, condition, or syndrome.[42]

---

* I first learned of the term "pregnant people" from abortion providers and staff at an abortion fund. It is the medically accurate term, as not all people who are pregnant are women, and not all women can get pregnant.

And despite the clear science linking polluted housing, alcohol exposure, and smoke—including secondhand smoke from someone other than the mother—to birth defects, the ghoulish, punitive, racist "fetal protection" crowd doesn't concern themselves with finding preventative solutions in those areas.

Then, of course, there's abortion. Abortion is essential medicine, simple to perform chemically or through a basic medical procedure. It's about 14 times safer than giving birth,[43] and significantly safer than carrying an unwanted pregnancy to term.[44] Yet getting an abortion requires navigating a mass of regulations insane in proportion to its ease and complication rate. I can't think of a similar instance of so simple a medical procedure so aggressively complicated by policy. This policy is, of course, intentionally designed to restrict access to abortion and other reproductive services.*

The game has been rigged such that people who need abortions suffer exponentially as the restrictions fold in upon themselves—the Hyde Amendment prohibits federal funds from being used on abortion services, which disproportionately affects pregnant people who don't have insurance or whose insurance doesn't cover abortion and thus might need financial assistance to get care.† These people are more likely to be poor. At the same time, Targeted Regulation of Abortion Providers (TRAP) laws are very narrow provisions that target abortion

---

* People who need abortions aren't the only ones who suffer from abortion restriction. Giving hospitals the ability to refuse performing surgery because of religious preferences leads Catholic hospitals to deny miscarriage management to pregnant people. Sometimes patients have to wait until they're in critical condition, bleeding out at the door, before the hospital will intervene. Great job, Catholics.

† The movement that will win single-payer will be the movement that repeals the Hyde Amendment. Otherwise, the resulting program will not be single-payer. (There are efforts in both the House and Senate bill to exempt the single-payer from Hyde, which seems like an acceptable intermediate step to me.)

clinics and impose excessively onerous and expensive requirements upon them—requirements more stringent than those
placed on other medical clinics performing more complicated
procedures. Clinics close, and some patients have to travel
hundreds of miles to seek help. These people, again, are more
likely to be poor.

That these are the two readily apparent consequences of
sexism in healthcare is a complication from a deeper injury:
womanhood, and the genre of "women's health," has been
reduced to one's reproductive capability—one's "usefulness."
This reduction is a massive act of structural violence, the
consequences of which can be witnessed in other kinds of
health inequity: for example, medicine optimized for men
just doesn't work quite as well on women. Women (and non-
binary and trans people) are historically underrepresented
in clinical trials, leading to both a higher rate of adverse
side effects when taking pharmaceuticals[45] and worsened
outcomes when treated with procedures that were tested
disproportionately on men.[46]

Of course, these structural forces don't ride alone. Women
and transwomen are disproportionately poorer than men, and
thus more dependent on social programs for their access to
healthcare.[47] Poverty is feminized.

POVERTY

Sometimes, when a politician feels bad about poverty, they'll
talk about "socioeconomic status" and how health outcomes,
etc., differ by it. This is like saying that health outcomes differ by "race" without specifying that racism is, in fact, forcing
the difference—it confuses the smoke for the fire, and presumes that some portion of the whole explosion is inevitable.

The construction of socioeconomic status disguises its composite categories, chief of which is income. When somebody is of "low socioeconomic status," it almost always means they're poor.

Poverty is complex, but it's not complicated. Poverty happens to most Americans at some point in their life—it is not an impermeable caste of Americans, but a cycle into and out of which people dip, sometimes multiple times a year. The cause of poverty is, of course, not having enough money. It can be caused or exacerbated by not having food, housing, or healthcare, which have their own causes and concurrences, like sexism and racism—all of which, in turn, deprive a person of the ability to make money. That is to say, not having money usually means you won't make money. Acquiring money is contingent upon having the ability to contribute your body or your wallet to the American economic sphere.

The invention of "socioeconomic status" ignores (or is not capable of understanding) that this is not something that happens accidentally. God did not shake the Earth like a snow globe and let the pieces fall as they may, determining in God's infinite wisdom that some people should lack what they need, while others swim in it a hundred million times over. That money was taken from some people and given to others. This is not a question of "poverty" as much it is one of *impoverishment*: people are not inherently poor; they're made poor.

When a growing amount of wealth is hoarded by a shrinking number of people, most of us can draw a connection between poverty and illness from somewhere in our own lives. So instead of pointing out the minutiae within "poor people are sicker than wealthy people," let's talk briefly about two groups completely shunned from the American economic sphere in different ways, and the extreme depravity of their health outcomes: Native Americans and transgender women of color.

Native Americans

Native Americans have been massacred and forcibly relocated into reservations across the United States—reservations often chosen because the land was not profitable to American farmers.* This extreme violence, now transformed into economic and racial segregation disguised as some sort of American benevolence, has crippling health consequences: in many states, Natives live 20 years shorter than non–Native Americans on average.

Some of these reservations are more remote than others, where echoes of past violence ring louder. The Rosebud Sioux reservation in southern South Dakota sits on a patch of land you might generously describe as "the middle of nowhere." There are few jobs, substandard housing, and high school graduation rates under 60 percent. Average family income is $18,000 a year,[48] less than a quarter of the 2016 American average family income of just under $80,000.

American life expectancy for men is about 79 years. But on the Rosebud reservation in southern South Dakota, male life expectancy is 47 years.[49] Since the introduction of the European to the American continent, Rosebud Sioux lifespan has dropped—almost by *half*—while lifespan of the European colonists and their descendants has more than doubled. Young adults on the Rosebud reservation aged 15 to 24 commit suicide at almost three times the rate of the rest of the teenaged American population.

---

* *Indian Reservations in the United States*, Laus Frantz, page 178: "For many years the federal government tried to make yeoman farmers out of as many American Indians as possible . . . The policy that sought to make Indian people individualized, self-sufficient farmers was doomed from the start, since most of the Indian land is not suitable for agriculture without large capital expenditure, owing to unfavorable climatic conditions, poor soil, and inadequate supplies of water."

And when Natives do get sick, there aren't many resources available for them. The Indian Health Service (IHS) is under siege. The IHS ostensibly pays for Native care, but receives a set amount of money (also known as a "block grant") each year, regardless of how many people need healthcare. Money runs out. Since so many IHS hospitals are in remote areas, IHS has difficulty recruiting health professionals—those who do join usually work short contracts, or rotate through on J-1 visa programs.[50] Remote hospitals are often unable to provide help beyond primary care, so IHS has to contract with private specialists at rates Congress does not adequately fund.* Natives can theoretically leave the reservation for care, but many live in non-expansion states and are not eligible for Medicaid—or any help at all.

As a result, the amount of money spent on Native healthcare per capita is about a third of that spent nationally.† What care is provided is, frankly, lousy—in Rosebud, children have been born in bathrooms and heart attack patients have waited over an hour for care.[51]

Transgender Women of Color

Transgender women of color are subject to forces of racism, sexism, and transsexism. Pushed out of the mainstream eco-

---

*   "In FY 2013, IHS denied 146,928 eligible PRC [purchased and referral care] cases amounting to a total of $760.855 million in unmet need." National Congress of American Indians, Fiscal Year 2017 Indian Country Budge Request, http://www.ncai.org/resources/ncai-publications/08_FY2017_health_care.pdf.

†   "In 2014, the IHS per capita expenditures for patient health services were just $3,107, compared to $8,097 per person for healthcare spending nationally." Ibid.

nomic system, they are significantly more likely than cis women of color and white trans women to, at times, engage in sex work to obtain money, food, housing, clothes, or other necessary goods.[52] Deterred from engaging in the healthcare system by experiences with unhelpful or actively antagonistic healthcare providers,[53] over a fifth of transgender women in the United States have HIV, a rate 48 times higher than all adults of reproductive age.[54] Among the transgender women with new clinical diagnoses of HIV/AIDS between 2009 and 2014, half were Black and a fifth were Latina.[55]

Of course, there's a carceral element here. Under the pretenses of public health, 33 states prosecute people with HIV who knowingly engage in various behaviors that may potentially transmit, or are assumed to transmit, the virus to others. These laws typically don't take into account the use of pre-exposure prophylaxis or condoms.[56] At least 180 people were been prosecuted under these laws between 2008 and 2013, including countless arrests for low-risk actions such as consensual, protected sex, and negligible-risk actions, such as biting and spitting. These laws are both worthless from an infectious disease prevention standpoint and only serve to perpetuate HIV stigma and discrimination. Ten states go so far as to force convicted individuals to register as sex offenders, making it even harder to obtain gainful, stable employment.[57]

Transgender women of color living with HIV are therefore comprehensively excluded from the traditional economic sphere and face a high risk of incarceration every time they perform commercial sex work, but they have few other moneymaking alternatives available to them. That incarceration increases their health risks: not only may they lose access to crucial antiretroviral therapy (ART) for HIV and hormone therapies while incarcerated, but they may also be exposed to physical and sexual violence due to their gender identity, especially when housed in an all-male prison complex.[58]

The prisons are hungry for trans women of color. Vague municipal loitering laws give police officers license to profile, harass, "deface," attack, and arrest them under pretenses of a possible prostitution charge.[59] It doesn't take much. Some jurisdictions permit but a single condom wrapper to be used as "probable cause" for arrest—it even happened in San Francisco. In a 2012 report on this practice, Human Rights Watch found that transgender women were often harassed and arrested for carrying condoms, whether or not they were or had ever been engaged in sex work.[60]

So what do you do? You're damned if you do, damned if you don't. Don't carry condoms, and you're exposing yourself and others to significant health risks. Carry condoms, and you can get picked up—or worse. Police are six times more likely to assault transgender people of color than white cisgender individuals.[61] This is a tortuous, brutal web, a construction of pure injustice that preys on people already vulnerable to health injustice and exacerbates their suffering.

BABYLAND

These structural determinants converge in Babyland.

Memphis is the largest majority-Black city in Tennessee and, as such, is ignored or maligned by state policy-makers. It's a frequent target of punitive welfare austerity measures and mass purges of welfare rolls. It is also home to several nuclear waste dumps, pushed right up against the poorest neighborhoods. (Half the people in America who live near commercial waste facilities are people of color.)[62]

Conditions are so bad that the Shelby County health department now celebrates that the county's infant mortality rate is down to 9.3 per 1,000 births—still more than the rates of Finland, Japan, Norway, and Spain combined.[63] This being

America, Black families are disproportionately made to suffer those losses—in Memphis, 20 Black children died for every 1,000 live births as recently as 2003. Twenty! That's 2 percent of Black births! That statistic isn't just unimaginable in America; it's unimaginable, *period*.

Where do poor babies go where they die? For a long time they went to Babyland, a corner of the Shelby County public cemetery—a potter's field for children. They were put to rest in cramped rows below the earth, in unmarked graves a block away from a Walmart.

Or, at least, they used to be—because in 2014, Babyland filled up.

Poor Black children in Memphis die in such volume—America is *killing* the poor Black children of Memphis by poisoning their mothers and poisoning their homes so effectively—that we have run out of room for their bodies.

When children are dying in such volume that we dump them in a lot behind a Walmart, the fight for single-payer must also be a fight for something much greater than single-payer. It is an effort to demand in our world the health justice we have been denied. For decades, the inadequacy and naked incompetence of the private insurance model has been left unresolved, and like a wound it has started to rot. None of us are safe in our bodies, and the slightest crack can ruin you—and your children—for life. We have been atomized and isolated and made sick—we have been *immiserated*—by the snakes of structural poverty, by structural racism, by patriarchal domination. The people of America have been crippled by not only a corporatist healthcare model that extracts profit from us like oil, but a colossal machine that seeks to pump wealth from the powerless and give it to those already powerful.

And so when we fight for health justice, we all fight side by side. Because:

- Environmental justice is health justice.
- Economic justice is health justice.
- Reproductive justice—for people who don't want to reproduce, and for people who do—is health justice
- And justice for Black lives, justice for brown lives, justice for Native lives, justice for trans lives, justice for the lives of immigrants, justice for people in prison, and the well-being of all people, regardless of age, gender, race, or creed, is health justice.

This is not a call for charity. It is a call for returning to the people what has been taken from them. It is an effort to fight off the apocalyptic, death-loving monsters who will one day murder every single one of us—but who will set upon some of us sooner, and more savagely, than others.

Fuck 'em.

CAUGHT IN THE WEB: OUR EXPERIENCES WITH AMERICAN HEALTHCARE

The particular intersections of health inequity laid out previously are huge and horrifying. But health, while huge in its horror, is also intimate and intensely personal; we suffer snugly within its contours as if they were custom-tailored to us. What seems like a small or opaque policy tweak to one person can bring either salvation or damnation for another whose healthcare needs are fragmented or more severe. The horizons of health injustice are dramatically expanded beyond insurance for someone whose healthcare is denied them by the state, by the police, by unsafe housing, by deindustrialization, or by the looming menace of ICE.

It is better to hear these stories from the people who experience them instead of from my summarization. To this extent, for the next few pages I'm sharing some anonymized anecdotes I've collected about health, health justice, and the deprivation thereof, plus some of my own notes. Some of these stories are from people I know well; others are from acquaintances; others yet are from total strangers. A few come from in-person discussion; most I received from the storytellers themselves. I hope they are useful.

CHRONIC ILLNESS

Early in December of 2018, I received a notice from Aetna that they would no longer cover a treatment I've received every six weeks for the last seven years called IVIG. After five appeals they issued a unilateral decision that their denial was final and I could no longer appeal.

I live with what is known as an orphan disease, a condition that is so unique or rare in presentation that the patient population is often too small to warrant studies or disease-specific drugs. The basis for the insurer's denial was a presumption that we lacked proof of the drug's efficacy to my case

Before IVIG, attacks of my disease would cause blindness, joint swelling, pain, lesions, neuropathy, and tremors. I had no choice but to rely on dangerously high amounts of prednisone to stay alive. Long-term use of cortisol steroids is extremely dangerous and can cause critical loss of bone mass, adrenal failure, and death.

We then appealed to Shire, the drug manufacturer, who refused to provide financial assistance on the grounds that I did not have one of four conditions approved by the FDA for treatment with IVIG. The out-of-pocket cost would be $35,000 every six weeks. That's over $300,000 a year—for one medication. I have fallen through the cracks in a system that focuses more on cost-benefit analysis than patient outcomes, and my health is now rapidly declining.

Like many people with a chronic illness, advances in medicine mean that with the right treatment protocol, I can live a mostly nor-mal life. If my care is considered to be part of the profit-driven market, I will always be treated at best as a customer and at worst as a liability.

For those of us who have directly experienced the tremendous bur-den of the private health insurance model, it is obvious that we need to move to a single-payer system in the United States. When patients or allies get upset with the center-left's rhetoric of guaranteeing "af-fordable access" to healthcare instead of Medicare for All, we're not seeking a handout. We're fighting for our lives.

D. P., NEW YORK

As someone who was born with cystic fibrosis, a brutally aggressive respiratory disease, I am constantly being reminded of the market value of my own body. Some quick numbers: the primary specialty prescription medication I have to take in order to stay breathing costs $292,000 a year. The last time I landed in the hospital, the total bill for my five-day stay was $75,000.

I currently hold private health insurance through my job, so I'm not paying the full freight on these expenses. Instead, I have the privilege of paying about $5,000 a year rather than $500,000, effectively reimburs-ing my health insurance company for the service of enabling everyone else to profit off of my body. What a joy and a privilege it fucking is!

S. W., 28, NEW YORK

★   ★   ★

There is an irony here that D. P. is extremely valuable to Shire—but only if they can get Aetna to cover IVIG. Other-wise, they're cast out. This tug-of-war is lethal. No "affordable access" model would take care of D. P. They can't settle for anything less. And neither must we.

SURVIVORS OF VIOLENCE

My mother was a victim of domestic violence at the hands of my father. My siblings and I all experienced his abuse in one form or another. My parents divorced almost 20 years ago, but since my dad is middle-class and relatively put together and my mother is poor and mentally ill, he got away with continuing abuse long after the divorce using the courts, his money and resources. He was ordered to put us on his health insurance, as my mother had none and three out of the four kids were disabled. He would periodically stop paying child support or pull us off the health insurance for periods of time with no consequences. I was born with juvenile rheumatoid arthritis and uveitis, and without going into all the details, both conditions can be permanently disabling if not treated well, and this period of time where money and insurance were being taken away were years when my illnesses were very active.

It was a long time before my mother found a job with insurance so that I could be treated, but by that point the damage of having treatments interrupted had already been done. I won't ever know if being treated continuously would have prevented this, but I am now irreparably blind because my conditions got progressively worse and the damage became permanent. I have long since accepted and learned to cope with my blindness, but the years of suffering and time spent on vocational rehabilitation probably didn't have to happen if I'd gotten treatment. For comparison, my sister, who is six years younger with the same conditions, happened to be diagnosed after my mother found work with insurance and had steady and continuous treatment throughout her childhood and adolescence. She has 20/20 vision and minimal damage. A few years ago, when I was doing my clinical internship at a domestic violence agency in grad school, I learned that this is not uncommon with abusers after they no longer have physical access to their victims. Financial abuse and weaponizing health insurance was something I saw happen to many of my clients, and it was always devastating.

M. P.

★   ★   ★

Abusers will use any weapon available to them. American health finance hands them a big one: domination of a survivor (and their child's) healthcare. Often, people who endure domestic violence will stay in the relationship, or stay in the home, because they or their children are financially dependent on their abuser—especially if they have chronic health conditions. The only tool available to a victim is the court system—yet the carceral state is entirely inadequate to the task of addressing domestic violence. Rather, the carceral state being the primary recourse of the abused, and the reluctance of survivors to put their abusers in prison, gives the abuser even more tools of control, prolonging the suffering.

DISABILITY

Navigating healthcare in the States reminds me of navigating a church with my disability, especially those modern, contemporary ones, where the lights are turned low and the sound system is tight. I will literally be listening to church leaders open with their mission of inclusivity, while I'm searching for that specific space in the back of the church to sit. Behind rows and rows and rows of folks standing, I look at a sea of denim bottoms. I consider what it would be like if disabled people were part of the planning team. What it would be like if we were included from the beginning of the planning rather than being an afterthought?

Living with spinal muscular atrophy, a motor neuron disease from which my muscles are slowly wasting away, I'm regularly adapting to new physical strengths (or, rather, weaknesses). I have never been able to transfer myself from one position to another. I have never been able to break the seal of a water bottle and drink. I did, however, used to be able to flip my hair from one part to another or take a big ol' bite from a raw carrot. Both of these things are mine no longer. These physical weaknesses from this genetic autosomal recessive disease have honed my ability to find solutions and advocate. Of course, I have learned how to tell churches and leadership that disabled people need to be present when creating new spaces or modifying existing ones. Speaking about access is a daily conversation. However, having leadership listen is not often part of my experience.

Which brings me to why navigating healthcare in the States feels like having to sit in the back of the church. True, I would not be alive without Medicaid. Yes, Medicaid covers my price-gouged power rehab wheelchair, my cough assist machine, and my home-health aides. However, I would like to push us a bit further. I believe we can do better than covering these costs with Medicaid. Medicaid requires that I remain poor to qualify. I cannot be married and receive Medicaid. I cannot own a home or a car and have Medicaid. Also, I must have almost no personal savings. Because Medicaid is allocated by each state, it is not the same coverage from state to state, so in some states, folks with my same diagnosis are not even receiving home-healthcare aides and have to live in institution-like settings, in nursing homes, with little to no quality of life. What if we solved this? What if the disabled were not left out of decision-making about the things that affect our health, whether on the national level or even leftist circles? What if masses of temporarily able-bodied folks were comfortable with acknowledging they have no experience and or knowledge about disability rights? What if these able-bodied folks recognized their opportunity to pass the mic?

God would not want us excluding Jesus from His church if he were disabled and used a power wheelchair. God would not shun disabled to the back, behind everyone who's standing and listening to how Jesus wanted us to spread good news to the poor and sick.

We can actually spread the good news. We can include disabled leaders in creating policy, hire disabled campaign staff, create systems *that breathe into access beyond ramps. The disabled and chronically ill should not be set aside, especially in the wealthiest country in the world. We are a country where Amazon pays a whopping $0 in federal income taxes on $11.2 billion in profits. There are 45,000 people dying a year because they don't have insurance, and countless more insured people dying because these insurance companies are ruthless, denying medicine in this wealthiest country in the history of the world. Unimaginable. We need to tackle our current healthcare system, of profit motives, together. A single-payer system must include disabled people and include long-term care, a system of health justice, where disabled people can own a home if they so choose, be employed doing whatever dream job might be had, and be included in the communities they live in and love. We must prioritize our individual health, and the health of our neighbors over the corporate profits that continue to create greater wealth disparity and poorer health outcomes. We must prioritize healthcare as a right, not a privilege.*

F. P., 41, SOUTHWEST OHIO

★   ★   ★

It's not very difficult to listen to people with disabilities and build inclusive movements and inclusive healthcare structures. Failing to do so is a laziness and lack of imagination. Senator Bernie Sanders's original 2018 Medicare for All bill continued delegating long-term care to state Medicaid programs—if that were to pass, in that form, it would be a moral calamity. It only changed because of organized pressure from the left. Let this be a reminder to never grow complacent with the bills offered to us, and to forever demand the real thing.

RACE AND HEALTH

I am a pathologist who specializes in blood transfusion. Historic disparities in the donor base created a near-impossible situation for sickle cell disease. These patients depend on chronic transfusions, which cause a phenomenon known as alloimmunization. Alloimmunization makes them more vulnerable to fatal or debilitating disease complications (stroke, lung and liver failure, blood attacking itself, etc.) from incompatible blood they need to (potentially) save their lives. The "curative" bone marrow transplant or gene therapy is out of most of their means, not just the treatment itself but its chronic post-therapeutic management. And their lives are shortened by these stopgap dependencies: pain-drug dependency requiring detox counseling, and dependency on exorbitantly priced drugs to take iron away from their blood so excess iron doesn't kill them before the blood might. With no national donor registry—the Red Cross tries to make their own—they inevitably end up in under-resourced public hospitals that may not recognize their illness as what it is, and mistreat them, or let them scream in bed for days with intractable pain and keep them there for days with no end in sight to their admissions. Let's admit this: this disease, which is pretty common in multiple regions of the country, is nonetheless treated like an "orphan disease" by national agencies. You can guess why. Doctors know and despair.

D. C., 35, ATLANTA, GEORGIA

★　★　★

There are about 100,000 people with sickle cell disease. It disproportionately affects Black people, and 1 in 365 Black children is born with it.[64] Structural racism in healthcare goes all the way to the top and all the way to the bottom. People of color both receive less care and receive a greater amount of low-quality care. When a disease like sickle cell resides primarily in a racial minority, or when it affects a population that is not white and wealthy, it is given less attention and fewer resources. This negligence kills.

One step below the level of research, we find that 30 percent of doctors see 100 percent of patients of color. That is—70 percent of doctors treat only white patients.[65] This happens when, for example, a hospital moves out of an urban area with a higher ratio of minorities to the lily-white suburbs. Ostensibly, they do this because the higher uninsured rate in the city drives down the hospital's net reimbursement rates, though that's an insufficient argument. It's just another way to continue segregating healthcare.

OPIOIDS

This is my, Timothy Faust's, essay. I'm 30 years old in 2019, so of course I have friends who have died in the opioid epidemic. It is more unusual to hear a friend has purchased a home than to hear someone has OD'd. I understand the opioid epidemic, more so now than I did when I first took to the road, but it is overwhelming to confront it every day a few hundred miles apart, to hear the same stories—that someone was just out of rehab, that insurance cut them off from a full course of treatment, that someone had just lost a friend, that someone had just lost a sister, that someone had lost five friends just this year—in every city I visited. That people felt comfortable coming to me and telling me their stories, that they shared with me a vision of the better world, is an honor. But it was in Indiana that I cried.

Indiana is home to Scott County, which you might know as one of the few places in the United States with a new population-wide epidemic of HIV/AIDS.[66] We understand the causes:

- *One, pharma companies have pushed tamper-resistant pills to market, which can't be crushed and snorted. This doesn't do anything to curtail abuse and addiction,[67] but it does let a pharma company claim to take opioid addiction Very Seriously while renewing the patent for its cash crop.* If you're a person battling addiction, not being able to snort doesn't keep you from using. You just dissolve it in water and inject it (or turn to heroin or fentanyl instead).*
- *Two, then-governor Mike Pence shut down needle-exchange programs in the state. Needle drugs are for criminals, we're told, because they're illegal. Why should we spend money on criminals' healthcare?*
- *Three, the state of Indiana gutted, shut down, or restricted funding for community clinics and places like Planned Parenthood.*

Here're the breaks: if you're a person in Indiana battling opioid use disorder, tamper-resistant pills mean you're more likely to turn to needles. Except now it's hard to find a clean needle since the needle exchanges shut down, and the other clinics you might turn to for help are unavailable too. The results are grotesque in their predictability: more people get HIV/AIDS and hepatitis C.

But that's not where the story ends. We work hard to dehumanize people battling addiction, to deny them the basic decency of personal agency and context. But they have families; they have communities. I spoke with a friendly young man who worked in the school system in Scott County. The county is now home to a necropolity—*a mass othering, a people denied their humanity and rendered non-people, a people treated as a big mass of Problems, floating in and out of the jail system. It is not a county of the walking dead, but the walking dehumanized.*

---

*   This is grotesque in its similarity to how Purdue created OxyContin and its unprecedented marketing campaign only when its patent on MS Contin was set to expire.

Indiana has a very low property tax cap, which limits school funding, and it also has a robust school voucher program. Better-off families who didn't want their kids to attend school with the children of people with HIV/AIDS or people in jail or people who use opioids sent their kids—and their tax dollars—elsewhere.

The flight exacerbated the drought of public money in Scott County schools. Now the district has a disproportionate rate of kids with someone at home battling addiction or in the system, and less and less money to spend. That's fewer teachers, less food, and no mental health or guidance programs. The man I spoke with said you could spot a kid going through hell from a mile away—a kid with a parent in the system, a kid without support system . . . a child unmoored. But there was nothing they could do to help. There was no funding for breakfast or therapy or daycare. There just weren't any resources for the children of the necropolity.

And so Scott County schools saw an increase in child suicides.

TIMOTHY FAUST, 30, BROOKLYN, NEW YORK

★   ★   ★

We know the causes of the opioid epidemic: drug manufacturers have lied, cheated, and bribed to make sure their painkillers are sold as broadly as possible. Purdue Pharma lied to doctors, patients, and regulators to push OxyContin into as many hands as possible, and to be prescribed as strongly as possible. Purdue ignored all evidence of addiction until they were compelled not to by law.[68] These motherfuckers keep doing the *exact same thing* today: in January 2019 the CEO of Insys Therapeutics pled guilty to giving kickbacks to doctors who prescribed Insys's oral fentanyl spray—even to patients who didn't need it. The CEO personally pocketed a neat $3.5 million from this arrangement.[69] Insys *also* produced a motivational video parodying A$AP Rocky's "Fuckin' Problems" to motivate their sales staff to persuade doctors to prescribe higher (and more expensive) titrations of *fentanyl spray* to patients on pain medication. A vice president of the company even dressed up in a fentanyl mascot costume.[70]

Meanwhile, people are in jail, people are addicted to painkillers from manual labor jobs, people who have chronic pain can't get the medicine they need, and the Sackler family, who owns Purdue, are throwing $2,500-a-person wine soirees at art museums. It will take $183 billion just to stabilize what they've done to America and it's never going to happen unless we demand it.[71]

The current national response to the opioid epidemic takes a supply-side approach. Supply-side interventions primarily focus on where people get drugs from: individual dealers and, occasionally, institutional ones. Now hospitals are spending tons of money to build complicated data-science operations to analyze prescribing behavior, which will do very little except create a new list of names to arrest and prevent people who do need medication from getting it. People with burning, searing, endless pain who are denied opioid medication are just left behind, told to "tough it out" or hope (hope!) that they contract a disease that justifies the medicine they need.

In this reform model, cops are used as social workers—a match made in hell if there ever was one—and are sometimes sent door to door in neighborhoods with high rates of opioid use to see if they can "help." (It doesn't work.) Our approach just means we send a hell of a lot of people to jail—a playbook inherited from the racist War on Drugs—and it clearly doesn't work. Supply-side interventions send people to prison, but they don't stem the need for opioids. Removing individual "bad actors" won't make the problem go away: the pharma industry—or the cartel—will create supply if a demand exists. There are infrequently town "dealers"—people who sell drugs are often people who use them, or friends or family of the end users themselves.

Underpinning all of this is that, for a lot of people, selling opioids is a rational choice if there aren't other jobs available. When the dollar store a town over is the only place hiring, selling at least helps you keep the roof over your head. Deindustrialization is a risk factor in opioid misuse.[72] We've just decimated huge swaths of the country in the past 40 years and this is the consequence. We can't police our way out of it. We can only build.

So if you want to reduce opioid use and opioid dealing, address the foundational problems that make it rational in the first place. Decriminalize opioids and free people from jail. Shore up the robust and redistributive social spending required to give people ways to avoid poverty. If there aren't jobs, *make* jobs, and ensure nobody's ability to eat or live safely is dependent upon their ability to work. Finally, invest in the primary care and pain interventions that can be used to help opioid-dependent people, or that can help prevent people from becoming opioid-dependent. We know that patient-directed care—basically, involving the patient and their family in the decision-making about their own care—works.* We know there are alternate pain management therapies, or less addictive drugs, that a patient can use. We know we can invest in the things required to help keep people from being in pain in the *first* place. And only these options—these slow, challenging, empathetic options—might help us help all of America.

---

* Fucking duh! Of course it works! And this isn't a secret: every conference I've been to about opioids features a speaker on it. But it requires treating the patient as a person, and it requires compassionate labor, and therefore has yet to become fashionable among the higher echelons of health-policy people.

TRANS HEALTH

My trans brother and I grew up in a rural Californian county with very few dental providers. As a teenager, my brother had to go out of the county to get his wisdom teeth pulled because the one dentist who took our insurance refused to see trans patients.

A. A.

I have to receive my insurance from a combination of alternating Medicaid and the Obamacare exchange. Since I came out, I've had a harder time getting and keeping work. I'm so lucky that I have a skill I can do remotely as a freelancer; otherwise, I have no idea how I'd be able to survive as a trans person in a cis-male–dominated industry.

Just having the insurance doesn't mean things are easy, though. Every year I have to go through a new set of hoops just to get the medications I need. Receptionists and even doctors have misgendered me and even told me they didn't approve of my being trans while they were writing me prescriptions for the medicine I need. It's like the dentist telling you you're a bad person for having a cavity.

I know some people who take matters into their own hands . . . kind of a DIY transition culture with black-market hormones. I've managed to stay away from that, but I don't know what I would do if I couldn't work. This is not recreational healthcare. This is who I am.

C. H., 32, ILLINOIS

★　　★　　★

Health finance is not kind to trans people. The 2015 U.S. Trans Survey found that a third of trans patients had reported experiencing harassment from a medical provider.[73] In January 2018, Health and Human Services (HHS) announced the creation of a new Conscience and Religious Freedom Division, which is explicitly intended to help providers find ways to refuse to perform care for "religious reasons"—similar to how Catholic hospitals can refuse to provide contraception or perform abortions or miscarriage management. Trans people who live in more liberal urban areas might be able to find a provider they're comfortable with, but that's not the case for people living in rural or conservative areas. The fight for trans equity in healthcare therefore rides a similar, but not identical, highway as the fight for reproductive justice: both are harmed by patriarchal domination in health and health finance. Single-payer cannot solve these problems on its own, but it can guarantee that trans healthcare is free, and enforce existing prohibitions against turning away patients for reasons of trans identity.

MATERNAL HEALTH

For 12 years of my adult life I did not have health insurance, so the only time I had any medical care were visits to urgent care clinics or the ER for serious injuries. After I got married I was able to get on my wife's insurance. About 25 percent of her pay goes to cover our premiums, which don't seem to cover much, and we have what many people consider a "good" plan.

In 2015 we had a stillbirth. Everything in the pregnancy had been going normal, mother and baby were both healthy and happy . . . until they weren't.

The thing a lot of people don't understand is that a stillbirth isn't the same thing as a miscarriage. In many instances of miscarriage the woman may not require any hospitalization or greater care beyond some postpartum doctor visits. A——— had to give birth to a 4-pound, 2-ounce, 19-inch baby girl who just so happened to no longer be alive. You. Still. Have. To. Give. Birth. There is no light at the end of that tunnel. There will be no happy ending after the baby is born. A——'s body had to go from not being prepared for labor at all to ready to birth a baby before she went septic.

My wife was in the most painful, torturous labor for 60 hours. The baby was born, we avoided a cesarean. We held our daughter Emerson Lucille ("Emmy Lou" for short) before the nurses took her away to be prepared for the funeral home. We had her cremated and brought her home. We were living in complete despair despite the best efforts of our capable and loving support system.

A birth isn't cheap, a five-day hospital stay isn't cheap, all those drugs and tests aren't cheap. We spent five days in anguish and pain and terror contemplating how we would go on. After insurance we were about $6,000 dollars in debt. Our daughter died and we had to pay for it.

A—— was back at the job one month later. Every day she had to go into that office and relive that moment until she couldn't anymore and quit to go back to retail.

It's been three years and Emmy has a little sister now. We made a ton of extra appointments to make sure we didn't have a repeat of last time. That was costly: insurance determined that a lot of those visits weren't necessary, and wouldn't cover them. The health debt hasn't stopped following us. We recently tried to get financing for a home loan so Emmy's little sister can have a place to grow up, but that medical debt was like a Molotov cocktail to our credit scores.

I know there're a lot of people who have it worse. We're doing pretty good, all things considered. But it still doesn't make it okay that all of us have to live inside this relentless meat grinder with no reprieve or early release for good behavior.

C. B., 33, AND A. B., 29, CHICAGO, ILLINOIS

★　★　★

My heart hurts. There are about 25,000 stillbirths a year in America, representing about 1 percent of all pregnancies.[74] Up to 20 percent of additional known pregnancies end in miscarriage.[75] Reproductive justice is for people who *want* to reproduce as much as it is for people who don't, yet America utterly devalues a willingly pregnant person once their pregnancy is ended. To hit the grieving family with five or six figures in medical bills is beyond barbaric—it is cruel.

MEDICAL COSTS

I grew up in pretty severe poverty and was lucky enough to have CHIP until the day of my high school graduation. My household had way too many people, and most of my family was severely toxic and difficult to live with. I lived a life similar to those you might see in "inspirational education movies," in that I tried to work fairly hard in school to avoid my family and my home. As a kid I was diagnosed with ADHD, something that my mother kept secret from me, as she didn't want me taking stimulants. This made it so that, despite high test scores in school, I constantly failed because I couldn't focus long enough to do homework.

Things got tougher in my early teenage years, when I was diagnosed with Marfan syndrome [a rare genetic disorder affecting the body's connective tissue]. I spent a year of my life taking significant amounts of school off to get poked and prodded and tested to ensure the diagnosis. Although it didn't affect my health directly at the time, it added on to the frustration and sadness I had felt already because of my poor grades in school. This is when the mental health kicked in, something that my grandmother (a sole force of good holding my insane family together) recognized and wanted to help me with, but as a 17-year-old I feared the stigma and didn't want to do anything.

Flash forward to my high school graduation. I lost my insurance the day I graduated, which didn't seem like much at the time. I was very ready to escape my house, filled with too many people and too many scary ideologies, so I moved out to the city a month after graduating without a job and without a penny to my name beyond first month's rent.

I had miraculously been admitted to my state college on the recommendation of a few teachers who really liked me, despite having a 2.0 GPA and barely (and I mean barely) finishing my credits in time. My time at school allowed me to see student clinic doctors when I could afford the co-pay, which wasn't often. I recall a time during winter break of my freshman year when I developed a severe and painful infection in my throat; I ended up getting in touch with a friend's mom who was a gynecologist to ask her for recommendations on low-cost healthcare in the area. Instead of recommending a clinic, she wrote a prescription for me that cured it within days. Without insurance, the drug cost me $94.

Soon enough I dropped out of college because I still couldn't focus on homework. Things were exceedingly difficult and my mental health got worse and worse in the years following. I managed to discover my ADHD diagnosis right before I began attending a semester at my community college, which was an absolute lifesaver. Medication and therapy helped, but not quite enough. The medication my nurse practitioner thought would be the best cost almost $200 a month without insurance.

On top of all of this, I had gone half a decade without any sort of checkup on the symptoms of Marfan syndrome. About a year ago I got a delirious fever and was rushed into the ER of a local hospital. Because of the Marfan, the doctor thought I'd had a lung collapse. Thank god, I didn't, but it was a virus that evolved into a severe and dangerous form of tonsillitis. I saw three doctors before anyone took me seriously. Two more prescriptions, two more ER visits.

Less than a year ago, due exclusively to health problems and financial struggles caused by them, I was right on the edge of killing myself. I ended up in the psych ward for a week, which was a wake-up call to those around me about the severity of my condition, but the stay itself didn't end up doing much. A week isn't enough time to tell. I spent the whole of 2018 seesawing back and forth between stability and absolute chaos.

I ended up meeting a nurse practitioner, through my grandmother, who has been a godsend. Her co-pays are $75 a visit, which is extremely straining on my wallet, but worth it in the end. Through her, we've sorted out my brain back to a point of relative functioning. I work two jobs now, at the city library and teaching private music lessons. I take three medications a day, with several more on hand as needed. With the help of [drug coupon website] GoodRx, I pay $103 a month to stay stable. At my last visit, they forgot to include the discount, and one of my prescriptions rang up as $550—for a 30-day supply.

My medical debt is crushing me. Despite relative stability, I can't imagine a foray further into adulthood (I am nearly 24 now) with any sort of success. I'm horrified.

And I'm in the [Medicaid] gap. Every year since the ACA was instated, I've been told that I make too much for Medicaid, but I can't afford any other plans. It is ruining me.

W. M., 24, SALT LAKE CITY, UTAH

★   ★   ★

If you can't afford healthcare, you don't seek healthcare. It's open-and-shut. If you don't seek healthcare, you get sicker. Why punish people with long-term consequences because they aren't profitable enough to take care of? W. M. didn't do a goddamn thing wrong except be born unlucky.

There's a legal theory of "financial toxicity," which I like a lot. It posits that the consequences of medical costs and medical debt are themselves a medical symptom—debt is stressful and incentivizes people to avoid seeking follow-up or further care—

and is one that doctors should be aware of.[76] Doctors are thus coerced to choose between providing someone with the care they need but can't afford, or the inadequate care they *can* afford. Either way, they're being compelled to harm their patients.

ABORTION

In my final year [of college] I had less than a thousand dollars to my name and got pregnant. I couldn't tell my family. I could count on one hand how many people I told for the first few years. I was on birth control, but I missed some days. I was in a long-term relationship with a partner I would stay with for the better half of that decade. I did everything "right," and I was deeply ashamed I let this happen. I dropped out of school.

I've spent the bulk of the last decade in therapy and now, at 30 years old, I have more medical debt paying for therapy and also student loan debt for my unfinished degree. Financial insecurity is trauma. I have been traumatized by my debt. Universal healthcare and-or free education would have changed my world.

I desperately want to be a mother someday. The only reason I am not is that I knew at 20 what I know still at 30, which is I can't afford to raise a child well with my current financial burdens. I am insecure and it's paralyzing. Reproductive justice is about being able to have or not have a family, and to have the resources for making that family well. I hope to still one day have children and I am utterly heartbroken that I lack the means to do that.

T. K., 30, PENNSYLVANIA

★   ★   ★

The football of abortion has been passed around on the single-payer debate until recently. Last year, the House "Medicare for All" bill, H.R.676, didn't even include abortion services. This is silly. Abortion is healthcare as much as a tonsillectomy is healthcare. Abortion happens regardless of whether people have "affordable access" to it—it just might not be safe. It is wielded like a club in the so-called "culture wars," but the only people who are dying are pregnant people who can't get the healthcare they need.

IMMIGRANTS

My very large family is mostly Vietnamese immigrants. Though they are lawfully present in the United States, at times it feels almost impossible for them to get the healthcare they need. Without knowing much English or having any connections, they are forced to work in minimum-wage (or, for the nail salon workers, sub-minimum) jobs without any benefits. Most of them aren't eligible to receive Medicaid until they've lived in the United States for five years.

My aunt works seven days a week in a nail salon and is splitting her blood pressure pills to make them last longer. On occasions when she has been afraid of running out, my dad has given her his own blood pressure pills. My cousin was born with Down syndrome—her parents can't afford Marketplace insurance, but they make too much to receive Medicaid where they live. My grandmother had an infection earlier this year that required short-term nursing home care. We were all nearly in tears when we learned that due to cost and location, our only option was a one-star nursing facility.

It isn't lost on me that anyone in the United States could have these health experiences. But my beloved immigrant family is navigating a racist, xenophobic, incomprehensible health system that only values them in dollar amounts. They have done every-thing this country has asked of them: they have jobs, they pay taxes, they are legally present, they send their children to school, they try to learn English. What does it say about our country and our policies when, even then, they can't access even basic medical care?

A. S.; 27, OKLAHOMA

★   ★   ★

Noncitizens face both active discrimination in healthcare as well as a higher uninsurance rate than citizens.[77] Hispanic children have the highest uninsurance rate (8 percent) of any ethnic group. We also know that mixed immigration status homes have very low insurance rates (certainly having to do with active disenfranchisement efforts both inside and outside healthcare).* As A. S. shows, immigrants are often excluded entirely from healthcare in America.

POVERTY

I am a severely physically disabled (Ehlers-Danlos and POTS) trans woman who has suffered with homelessness on and off. Healthcare is entirely inaccessible to me without insurance, which is inaccessible to me without a job that provides it (because Medicaid expansion was not approved here, and I cannot work because of the severity of the disability) or without the insurance provided by Disability Assistance (and I cannot get approved for SSI [Supplemental Security

---

*   We also know that we can significantly improve insurance enrollment rates by sending social workers to train Spanish-speaking mothers of insured children to help enroll their communities. Community movements work!

Income] because they require extensive documentation from doctors and physical therapists, something that would cost me tens of thousands of dollars to obtain without insurance). Instead, I have been forced to couch-surf and survive off the charity of friends for the past eight years.

C. S.

I am a type I diabetic. The way we are treated in this country is tragic. My fiancée was promised health insurance at a new job and for six months has been told they're "working on it." Luckily (as sad as it may seem) my mother is also a type I diabetic. I get my insulin from her, my syringes from an online store, and my test strips from Kroger. I am going to die eventually from this disease, and the most crushing part is that I know it won't really be the disease that has killed me, but poverty.

Diabetes is something that has been monetized, like a cable bill. Except if you don't pay that cable bill, you die.

D. R.

★   ★   ★

We anchor whether you're allowed to exist in your body to whether you make somebody else rich. You don't just need to spend money to make money; sometimes, you need to spend money to be able to afford not having any money.

Poverty doesn't just happen to people. They are made impoverished by a society that could prevent the problem but instead continues it—*deepens* it—all so some can profit while millions suffer.

MENTAL HEALTH

I have an invisible disability, or at least it's a disability by the standards listed on one of the last pages of any job application. I want to believe the truth of my answer, that I do have major depressive disorder, will not count against me, especially as I apply for jobs in the world of public health, where access for those with chronic illness is a huge component. But with shame and fear, I often deny I have any disability, or I mark that I do not want to answer at all. I want to believe that my ability to complete a job does not have to be hindered by the grogginess and sadness and sudden crashes of energy. I have had depression for more than half my life, and anxiety for the past 10 years. I hide it well. Just as I was nearing the commencement ceremony of graduate school a few years ago and as I frantically applied for jobs to companies that never responded, I had a major depressive episode. I was put on an antidepressant and enrolled in a partial hospitalization outpatient program for 10 days, where I was able to come out from under the fog of listlessness little by little. But when my student insurance ended by the end of that summer, I was abruptly cut off from seeing the therapist who had been key to my recovery, and if I wanted to see my psychiatrist, I was to pay out of pocket. That American health insurance is at all tied to whether one is employed keeps me at a disadvantage. Without insurance, I have to take bare minimum measures to stay afloat. Without a job, I cannot pay for any additional care I may need in the future. Being at my healthiest is imperative to performing well enough for a job interview, and overcoming my anxiety is crucial when networking is generally how people bypass electronic job application portals. I am in a bind and I keep it to myself. I am highly educated and highly qualified, but I am also sick and poor. I have never told an employer in the public health field about my health, because as long as I keep up the act, the depression is unseen. I do not know what I would do if I was suddenly stuck with a physical disability like blindness, or an expensive illness like cancer. I morbidly joke with my boyfriend and friends that if I'm ever in a serious car accident to just let me die because one ambulance ride and one emergency room bill would bankrupt me and lead to years of ruined credit. I joke that if I'm ever admitted to the hospital that I should just be killed immediately, as every day spent as an inpatient is thousands and possibly hundreds of thousands of dollars I do not have. I do not know if a person's life should have a price tag, but it doesn't include the hidden costs of shame and stigma.

D. S., 30, VIRGINIA

★   ★   ★

There's a joke that public health degrees are the only degrees you get so you can make *less* money than whatever you made before. What a bitter irony that students of health policy are often the ones who are most trapped in the web of restrictions, networks, and deprivation spun by the hegemonic corporate private insurance industry.

PROVIDERS

As a provider in an underserved community, one of the most frustrating things is seeing how underinsurance or lack of insurance really impacts your day-to-day life. The obvious example of medical bills aside, there are so many patients for whom their insurance status forces them to reconfigure basic parts of their life. For example, I had a patient who had a deep vein thrombosis, the treatment for which is a minimum of six months anticoagulation. The standard treatment is heparin with a five-day stay in the hospital to transfer to the drug warfarin. Warfarin levels must be regularly monitored by blood draw, which requires regularly going to a lab. Newer drugs called direct oral anticoagulants (DOACs), such as Eliquis and Xarelto, don't require a five-day inpatient admission and do not require regular monitoring. However, this pa-

tient's insurance refused to cover DOACs, so he was stuck in the hospital for six days and is now on a drug that requires him to get weekly blood draws, which means he has to go to a lab during their operating hours, wait, get his blood drawn, and follow up the next day for results. If his insurance covered the DOACs, none of this would be necessary. The healthcare system sucks for so many reasons, but the physical drain it puts on people is staggering and we cannot be surprised when people stop seeking medical care due to exhaustion. I know I would.

J. E., NEW YORK, NEW YORK

★   ★   ★

I mentioned earlier that people of color, as well as poor people, not only get worse care, they get more *bad* care. This is etched into the design of their insurance plans. J. E. offers a clear example. A person had to stay in the hospital for *six days*, and now has to get blood drawn every week, all when another available drug could have prevented it.

Here we have the express preferences of both the patient and his doctor brusquely overruled by a private insurance company's desire to profit. This is a violation of the doctor-patient relationship. Private insurers can be no longer permitted to trample upon it.

WORK

Nowadays I fight wildfires. With a seasonal job, I change my insurance plan three times a year.

- *I get a new plan in January, usually Obamacare, if I qualify.*
- *In May, I can switch to government healthcare, which is kind of a zoo. From the FEHB (Federal Employee Health Benefits)*

*options, I pick the cheap NALC plan. (National Association
of Letter Carriers; the envelope has a note on the back for your
USPS carrier like "Protect this sacred paperwork; it provides for
your brethren!") My NALC plan is administered by Cigna.*

- *In October, fire season ends and I lose insurance. I have to choose
between three more options: go back to ACA, pay the government
plan myself in full, or just hope I stay healthy until New Year's.*

A lot of seasonals don't bother with summer insurance. In a 16-
hour workday, any injury while awake probably happens on the
clock, and goes to worker's comp.

Not my luck. One day after I returned from fire season 2017, I hurt
my back.

I discovered that even if I have coverage, I have no coverage. Three
new plans a year means paying the deductible three times. Most of
my physical therapy came out of pocket. Even still, I spent afternoons
on the phone with a notepad, getting shuttled between Forest Service
HR, FEHB, the NALC, and Cigna.

I could summarize the complicated weeds of my actual coverage. After my injury in October 2017, I hastily signed up for the COBRA equivalent, and kept that coverage through 2018. January 2018, deductibles
reset. In May 2018, when the Forest Service could pay for my healthcare
again, I had to reapply. Unbeknownst to me, they opened a new NALC
plan, took money out of my paycheck for it, and kept mailing bills for
the COBRA NALC plan. So I had two plans running in parallel.

I didn't notice. As soon as we went available, I spent 31 days
straight in Colorado, returned for two days of R & R, and went
straight to California. That schedule offered limited opportunities to
call acronyms and listen to hold music.

This off-season, I stayed uninsured until January. I'm honestly
not sure exactly where I stand with the bureaucracy. I refused to pay
them for the COBRA double coverage.

B. Y., 35, OREGON

My dad was let go from a job right before I was born because of my
hemophilia. To this day I fear even using my employer-provided in-
surance for my hemophilia.

T. C., 29, NEW YORK

★   ★   ★

This is the employer-sponsored insurance system that oppo-
nents of single-payer tell us Americans are so keen on keeping?
That we're afraid of introducing some friction to transition to
single-payer? There's already an unfathomable amount of friction—and none of it ever breaks in your favor.

There exists a strategy of organizing for single-payer by tar-
geting employers with promises of lower costs. That's probably
accurate—employers will not need to contract with insurance
companies and spend money on premiums—but I worry the
strategy is ineffective. How many employers out there are
looking for the legal loopholes that let them cut off a sick or
costly employee? How many employers relish the power they
have over a person's life or death, or their kid's life or death,
because of employer insurance?

No, I think single-payer represents a great unchaining of
the American worker: a chance to finally be able to quit a job
or organize your workplace without fear of employer domination over a sick husband or a sick kid.

PART VI:

WHAT WE DO

This can all feel like so much. It feels like so much to me! I sit to read or write and the waves batter me and my body feels like a towel, wet and crumpled on the floor; I fall inside myself and wish for some angelic comet to plunge into my house and gently, quietly lift us all from this national suffering. But I don't think that's fair of me to do. It's not very kind to indulge in nihilism when other people have even more at stake. What do you do? How do you tilt against the grotesque squalor of the world?

My answer begins with single-payer. Single-payer won't solve all of the problems we've talked about in the previous section of this book. It won't even solve most of them: it won't build the houses, it won't feed the people, it won't bring jobs or money back to rural areas. But that's all right, in a sense— no program can, not all at once. What single-payer *can* do, I believe, is serve as a ladder we can climb, all together, into a better world. A properly designed single-payer program is one titanic step toward making people safe in their own homes, in their own bodies. It is a reprieve from our continual fucking-over by the structure and stricture of private insurance. And it is a method of finally demanding accountability from a state that permits (or even encourages) the sins that cause mass suffering—and the medical inequities they produce.

It's not a hard sell. Single-payer isn't that complicated (the real complicated shit is the various bureaucratic coping mechanisms invented to respond to the inadequacies of private insurance!) and most people like it already. More people will be drawn to it once they learn what it means and how it fits into the nooks and crannies of their lives. Most doctors and nurses like it, both because they've seen the devastating consequences of uninsurance among their patients and because they'd like to avoid the grating bureaucracy of trying to get paid by insurance companies.

The people who tend not to like single-payer are people who wouldn't like anything that didn't make them money: the insurance companies it would replace, plus the pharmaceutical, device, and hospital CEOs whose profits might be cut into by the rise of a larger, stronger, payer. Then there's the powerful people who generally benefit from human suffering: the abusive boss who wants to make sure you can't quit your job; the abusive husband who wants to make sure you can't quit your relationship; the CEO who enjoys being able to cut benefits while knowing his workers can't strike for fear of losing insurance; the lizardlike politicians who find it useful to first advance policies that let rich people plunder their districts, then blame poor people, people with disabilities, and people of color for the resulting scarcity.

These problems are not new in America. We've been suffering needlessly for generations. We continue this suffering because, at every conceivable opportunity, our politicians, our policy-makers, the CEOs who mine us for profit—have decided to pursue moderate, subdued, pragmatic, and useless policies. They have had every opportunity to help and have refused. They must be left behind. They've started coming out of the woodwork, and they'll continue to do so for the next few years. They'll have "responsible solutions" for "new American healthcare." They'll smile and go on TV and say they're very concerned about all these problems whose structural causes they, personally, have benefited from. They will reach out to take our hands, tenderly and piously, and whisper, "This really is the best we can do right now," as they jam them in the garbage disposal. So they're out.

We will have to turn to each other.

WHAT HASN'T WORKED

There's a lot of history to learn from. The fight for single-payer (or, before any payers existed, universal healthcare) is not new—it's been running in parallel with the development of the entire insurance industry. Beatrix Rebecca Hoffman, a historian of healthcare inequity and healthcare organizing, wrote a wonderful brief history called "Health Care Reform and Social Movements in the United States."[1] I recommend it; she demonstrates *why* our healthcare movements thus far have failed. I would prefer not to fail again.

For the past hundred years, health reform legislation has been in many cases the domain of well-meaning, well-intentioned insiders. But every time these insiders—the senators, the policy-writers, even the union or nonprofit leaders—have taken on the insurance industry, they have been beaten by a reactionary establishment (described, unflatteringly, above) that is capable of outmaneuvering, outfoxing, and outgunning health reform. The establishment has money and power, and if you come at them from within, they can swat you down. The policy insiders and think-tank presidents have learned that they can write a healthcare bill and wave it around to gin up support among the grass roots, but they have lost, over and over and over again.

They lost in the 1940s by "discourag[ing] rank-and-file initiatives" and "never consider[ing] grassroots mass mobilization."[2] They lost in the 1970s, when, despite working with civil rights and antipoverty groups, the universal healthcare bill was drowned out by 13 competing bills sponsored by industry and establishment organizations.* They lost in the 1990s when the Clinton administration tried to assemble a huge, complicated series of public-private partnerships that would somehow try to keep everyone satisfied—except the grass roots, who either got confused by an incredibly dense policy† or were ignored when they demanded more. The Patient Protection and Affordable Care Act of 2010 was lauded as a massive success by a subsection of liberal commentators in its time, but . . . if it were *actually* successful, I wouldn't have to write this book.

Hoffman sees victory in healthcare reform coming from grassroots movements—she cites ACT UP as a prime example. ACT UP (AIDS Coalition to Unleash Power) is perhaps best known for their powerful, dramatic protests—throwing the ashes of their loved ones who had died from AIDS on the lawn of the White House. Here, in the relative comfort of 2019, it's hard to remember how completely marginalized people with HIV/AIDS were in 1987.‡ A sizable portion of the federal government actively ignored the epidemic, and explicit descriptions of it as a "plague from God" were tolerated, if not welcomed. ACT UP organized not just people with HIV/AIDS but formed coalitions with organizations of people of color, women, and people who use needle drugs (who were disproportionately likely to get HIV), and through years of collective effort forced mayors, presidents, and corporations to take action—and then, crucially, kept the pressure on after they got their initial goals.

---

* This is a reason why people who would like single-payer healthcare must, unfortunately, take things like "Medicare Extra for All" seriously; they must be summarily debunked and dispermitted.

† Foreshadowing the ACA? Maybe!

‡ I admit that it is even harder for me to remember 1987 because I was not yet born.

I would additionally cite ADAPT as a powerful popular health movement in contemporary times. ADAPT is a coalition movement for rights for people with disabilities. The fights they have had to take on just to be treated like people are *many*, from transit access to home health to the current fight for the Disability Integration Act. You might know them as the reason Medicaid still exists as it does today. During Congress's various ACA replacement debates, ADAPT protestors bused down to the Capitol and protested on the floor. They were arrested, their healthcare devices broken, and they were dragged screaming to police buses and hauled off to jail without care or concern for their medical needs. The next day, they came back—over and over and over again.

These grassroots movements have succeeded. While perhaps they haven't succeeded as much as they'd like to—these are literally matters of life and death—they've done more than any think tank in all the East Coast. But they cannot win what they deserve—what *we* deserve—alone.

We have an obligation. We must not lose again. We stand on the shoulders of hundreds of thousands of nurses, of tens of thousands of doctors, in the legacy of grassroots movements like ADAPT and ACT UP—and we must build the massive popular movement that not only demands single-payer from our government, but demands health justice in our nation.

The bill we need does not yet exist. There are bills that are good, there are even good single-payer bills, and though I hope they pass, they are not and will never be sufficient in and of themselves. Any health justice movement that is satisfied by an existing bill, or that organizes around a bill, instead of around and among the people who are most immiserated, will follow its historical predecessors and fail. It has already failed.

So the answer is easy: skip the politicians and go to where the people are. Because the people need help. And we have to do it together.

WHAT WILL WORK

Idaho hardly seems like the place for a health justice movement. It's an overwhelmingly beautiful place that holds some of the dream of the American Western frontier: a place you can go to get away from everyone else and, among the mountains and the forests, have some peace of mind. It is not so much conservative as it is isolationist (though the line between the two has narrowed in the past few decades). Its one metropolitan area, Boise, accounts for a little under half the state's population. The rest of the state sprawls northward, a composition of scenes of great beauty.

Amid this beauty there is, of course, deep and widespread suffering. Rural hospitals are particularly overwhelmed in Idaho, as a shriveling safety-net program saddles them with high costs and a mostly uninsured population. Some of them close. After the passage of the ACA the Idaho legislature refused to expand Medicaid for various reasons: a weak governor, a coalition of far-right politicians, general Democratic reluctance.

Then, in November 2018, a ballot measure to expand Medicaid in the state passed. And not by a little—with a 61 percent majority. It passed in four-fifths of the counties, not just in the urban areas.[3] There was no "blue wave" in the state—the Democratic candidate for governor lost by 22 points.

Medicaid expansion in Idaho took a form virtually unseen in contemporary America—or, at least, the America that matters to the pundit class. It was a popular movement built by constant, diligent labor: a hundred meetings, a thousand canvasses, a hundred thousand handshakes.

I spend a lot of time exploring the mass immiseration of people in America. I take a lot of steps in the shadows of the cruel and opulent machine. So I often seek a chalice to bear, and in Idaho I glimpsed a small and powerful hope.

The movement started when the northern Idaho ski town of Sandpoint refused to pass a tax to fund its schools. Idaho schools are notoriously underfunded after a decade of property tax decreases and education spending cuts. Three friends—Emily Strizich, her husband, Garrett Strizich, and Luke Mayville—had enough and decided to run a citizen campaign to pass a lien to keep their schools funded. It succeeded.

The movement grew. They called themselves Reclaim Idaho and, after driving around talking to people, they set their sights on Medicaid. Reclaim Idaho bought an RV, painted it green, and decided to keep driving—all across the state, talking to literally anyone they could. They found people who knew their communities and who would volunteer to organize them. Then they kept driving.

From this patchwork campaign Reclaim Idaho became a bona fide DIY statewide movement. While the three core Reclaimers coordinated resources across the state and put together hundreds of events, local organizers were generally trusted to organize their areas as they saw fit. Which they did: thousands of volunteers knocked, texted, and called hundreds of thousands of people. Events in virtually every county of the state brought elected officials, doctors, people without insurance, and other citizens together to talk about Medicaid. The proposition got on the ballot with plenty of room to spare and not much money spent. The creaky state Democratic party alternately shied away from and then glommed onto the movement, depending on whether they thought it would poll well.

The Reclaim Idaho volunteers I met spoke of kindness, of fairness, and of economy. They went to their neighbors in urban areas, in rural ones, in trailer parks, in the sticks, in gas stations and grocery stores and college campuses. They spoke about how Medicaid expansion was free federal money to help people who are suffering, which would then be invested in Idaho's medical workers. They shared stories of making too much money to qualify for Medicaid and falling in the gap, they talked about rural hospitals that couldn't afford to treat their uninsured patients, they talked about the parts of Idaho that were ravaged by uninsurance. They talked about justice.

And then the people turned out to vote and extended the basic decency of healthcare to their neighbors.

The three Reclaim Idaho founders insist that this was not their movement alone. It was a campaign they coordinated, but it was funded and powered by normal people trying to pitch in and help, a banner carried by thousands of volunteers every single day until the last minute, a thousand torches held aloft in a great and spectacular line from the forest to the mountains. I watched a Reclaim volunteer run into a small dive bar and canvass everyone there with about 15 minutes before polls closed. He succeeded and escorted one young voter to the polling station two blocks away. "I didn't want to leave anything on the table," he told me.

And the whole thing was so damn wholesome. I saw grand-parents, grandchildren, friends, neighbors, and kids—every-one working together to feed each other, take care of each other, nourish and support each other, as they all sought to reach out and find new people to speak with. Like many folks my age, I've kind of self-atomized: I've never been close with my family; I'm never having kids; I move from city to city like a traveling circus. I like the family I have constructed for myself. But it really does feel special, safe, and nourishing to watch an extended community-family take care of itself. It is the self-regenerating model by which a larger one can be, slowly, and with difficulty, constructed.

There were but minutes between the news that Medicaid expansion had passed and vows from Republican lawmakers that they'd find a way to gut it, or attach work requirements. This would not be permitted. Reclaim Idaho mobilized the same people who came out to pass the bill, and they defended it—calling drives, rallies, protests. Candidates who did not win in November came out to train volunteers to effectively petition their representatives. There were more potlucks, more cookouts, more movements. In January 2019, Idaho Proposition 2 was signed into law. In February, the state submitted a Medicaid expansion request to CMS.[4]

I insist that this is the model—this is the only model—by which health justice can ever be realized in America. Lovingly, devoutly, and diligently—an organized, focused, and trusting movement building community for those who have most been harmed—borne from the specific furies of love. All your lightning waits inside you.

We must extend the basic decency of "showing up"—going to the people around us, listening, asking questions, finding common ground, and putting our shoulders to the wheel. We must identify what battles we can win, and then win them. We must provide material relief for the people around us who are suffering now.

We must fight in our homes for a continuous spectrum of demands aimed toward health justice. Unlike liberal policy-tweak incrementalism, our successes must be material and redistributive reforms. We must bring to the front our neighbors and friends who have been made to suffer most cruelly, and we must demand that the crowns of thorns thrust down upon their heads are lifted. We cannot rest until they are liberated from the suffering inflicted upon them.

We don't have to start from scratch. People have been fighting injustice much longer than any of us have been alive. We just have to show up.

In San Francisco, a coalition won Prop F, the right to counsel for people who are evicted.* In Maine, the Maine People's Alli-

---

* Part of this coalition was the SF Democratic Socialists of America, who are wonderful. They also beat a proposition that would give the police more funding (to be used on Tasers). Beating the landlords and the cops at the same time is a hell of a résumé.

ance won a significant minimum-wage campaign at the ballot box in 2016. They then turned out their volunteer base for the minimum-wage campaign to collect signatures to put Medicaid expansion on the ballot—which they did, very quickly, and then won again in 2017.* In San Antonio, the movement for paid sick leave collected 144,000 signatures—40 percent more than the number of people who voted for mayor in the previous election, making it the largest popular movement in San Antonio in years, if not decades. A couple hours north, in Austin, where barely anybody can afford to live anymore, a coalition of grassroots activists won a $250 million affordable housing bond at the ballot—more than twice the sum of every other housing bond in city history.

There are setbacks. Each of these victories can be waylaid by a malicious politician. But I think these victories are building blocks. If we give people something material, they will fight to keep it. If we fight with people today, they will fight with us tomorrow. We build solidarity so that we can build power. Our job is not to build one massive popular movement. It is to *stitch together* a popular movement—a big, messy quilt of movements for health justice at home, spanning the country from coast to coast and plains to gulf.

This is all to say that the work of health justice is not siloed. Housing work, healthcare work, anti-carceral work, disability liberation—all share health equity in their articulations of a better world. This and only this, I think, can bring about single-payer, and, beyond it, health justice. We have seen that movements for universal healthcare that are led from the top down have not succeeded.

Yet through this massive mobilization—and only through

---

* Maine Governor Paul LePage, a bloated tumor stuffed into a suit jacket who destroyed the state's Temporary Assistance for Needy Families program, ignored the ballot initiative and it wasn't signed into law until his successor, a Democrat, took office in 2019.

this massive mobilization—this is a fight we will win. Single-payer is *already* a wildly popular idea among the people it affects. This is not a radical proposition. We are simply discussing a basic principle of fairness.

After all, we all come from nothing. We are all fashioned from a formless and shapeless place. We have been thrust through the maw and born into a world that is arbitrary and unequal in its allocation of suffering. And yet instead of affording each other the basic dignities of being human, we have developed this bizarre system of American health in which one's suffering is one's own responsibility, in which empathy is vestigial and unnecessary. We have atomized suffering and, in turn, assigned blame for suffering to the people who suffer it.

I have seen such naked suffering inflicted in my American name. I have seen neighborhoods ripped apart by the unrepentant, unyielding bloodlust of capitalism. I have seen families torn limb from limb in the service of extracting profit. I have seen the dehumanizing machine all at once and felt despair. For me it is heinous to feel complicit, through my simple existence in my only and horrible home, in the mass immiseration and annihilation of those against whom the whole rotten weight of the world is stacked.

This is intolerable to me. I hope it is to you, too. And so I hope you join me in saying: enough. Not in our name may this America persist. May we root ourselves not in fear but in love—love for those who suffer around us, as we, too, will one day suffer—and from that love, may we cultivate the fury by which this cruel machine can be destroyed.

My friends—single-payer is moral. Single-payer is necessary. Single-payer is achievable. Solidarity now, solidarity forever.

AUTHOR'S NOTE

Flip back to the cover of this book. Do you recognize the symbol used in the background? It's two snakes wrapped around a staff. To many Americans, this is the symbol of health, medicine, and healing.

Except that's not quite what this symbol represents. The ancient Greek symbol of healing is actually the staff of Asclepius, a wandering healer who eventually became the god of medicine. His staff has only one snake wrapped around it. It is the staff of Hermes which features twin snakes, and this staff (the "caduceus") is a symbol of commerce, merchants, and thieves. The confusion between these snake staves—one virtuous, one vicious—is uniquely American, and dates back to the early twentieth century, when the US Army Medical Corps chose the caduceus as its logo.

This isn't an especially niche complaint. People who practice medicine seem to be aware of it well enough: a majority of professional medical associations use the one-snake symbol, while a greater majority of commercial organizations and large hospitals use the two-snaked staff.* It's a small difference, but it really gets my goat. Over the past century, we've venerated a symbol of deceit and theft and called it medicine. In parallel, we've handed the keys to the American health

---

* See Friedlander, Walter J. *The Golden Wand of Medicine: A History of the Caduceus Symbol in Medicine.* Contributions in Medical Studies, no. 35. New York: Greenwood Press, 1992.

system to a bulging mass of scammers and profit-seekers; the various corporations of American health finance. Is this not perverse? We have ceded even the basic iconography of health to those who wish to make money off of us. We've gone ahead and mistaken *commerce* for *care* in both the symbolic and the actual performance of medicine

What a lousy trick! But numbering the snakes is just tapping away at a very small tip of a boat-annihilating iceberg. It is my hope that this book may help you see more of the full-body bamboozlement of American health finance, and that it may furthermore help you understand how a gentler world is possible.

★   ★   ★

There's only so much you can cover in 60,000 or so words. That said, I've tried to do my best to incorporate both the important popular facts about single-payer as well as the broader ecosystem of health and health justice, but there's certainly important stuff I didn't cover. If you have questions, I encourage you to sign up for my newsletter (http://www.tinyletter.com/error) and search the archives. If you can't find it, you are more than welcome to email me directly and I'll get back to you within a couple of weeks. My email address is tim.faust@gmail.com.

If you want to learn more about American healthcare, here are some good things to read.

- *Health Care at Risk*, by Timothy Jost
- *Health Care for Some: Rights and Rationing in the United States Since 1930*, by Beatrix Rebecca Hoffman
- *Fixing Medical Prices: How Physicians Are Paid*, by Miriam Laugesen

- *Medical Apartheid: The Dark History of Medical Experimentation on Black Americans from Colonial Times to the Present*, by Harriet A. Washington
- *Poverty and the Myths of Healthcare Reform*, by Richard Cooper
- *Poor People's Movements*, by Frances Fox Piven
- *Killing the Black Body: Race, Reproduction, and the Meaning of Liberty*, by Dorothy E. Roberts
- *Health Affairs* journal. It is accessible, nicely designed, and a pleasure to read. The March 2018 issue is a personal favorite.
- The writing of Tim Jost, Uwe Reinhardt, and PNHP's Don McCanne
- The journalism of Libby Watson (currently at Splinter), Jeff Stein (at the *Washington Post*), and Dylan Scott and Sarah Kliff (both at Vox)

ACKNOWLEDGMENTS

There are too many people to thank and I'm dreadfully afraid of leaving anyone out. It takes a village to raise a child, and I weigh as much as at least three children.

Steve Way and Kyle Kolich reached out to me with a wrestling offer I couldn't refuse, and have since become friends, teachers, comrades, and a source of endless videos of Bret Hart.

Everyone who submitted a story for the micro-essays on the intersections of health shared a deep part of themselves with me, and I am so grateful and so moved by your empathy and generosity.

My friend Jen McKinney; my mentor, friend, and de facto older brother Mateo Hoke; and my best friend, Krista Ziegler, read this book and gave me compassionate, critical feedback. Brandy Jensen found ways to pick me up when I was afraid I had fallen down. Frank Firke, Kate Hildebrandt, and Ankit Kumar have been wonderful people and very game to answer my healthcare questions, tell me a story, or point me to resources. Nate Martinez read my manuscript, sent me hours of reading about race and health, took me on a driving tour of Bridgeport, Connecticut, introduced me to mofongo, my new favorite food, and became my friend. Virgil Texas, Matt Christman, Felix Biederman, and Will Menaker first gave me a platform and helped me realize I liked talking about healthcare. My dad, Big Jim Faust, once drove twelve hours in three days to see my same speech three times and give me a break from the road, which at the time was the nicest thing anyone could ever do for me.

Emily and Garrett Strizich and their family took me in for a week and let me watch them work, winning Medicaid in Idaho. I've never felt such ecstasy and hope after an election.

I spent much of 2017–2018 on the road, talking to people about healthcare in their homes. I've met hundreds of people and spoken to thousands, and each one of them gave me a little something that I tried to let shine in this book. To you who took me into your homes, gave me your beer and your spare beds or couches, who came up to me after a talk and told me your stories—thank you.

Ryan Harrington and Alex Primiani, my editor and publicity director respectively, and the rest of the team at Melville House were ceaselessly gracious, accommodating, and shockingly chill as this book came together, then fell apart, then came together again . . . a few times. Thank you for taking a chance on an unknown author.

Most importantly, I would like to thank my partner, Kelly Jo Popkin, to whom this book is dedicated. Too many male authors have coasted upon the work of their girlfriends and wives and given them no credit. With them in mind I endeavored to do this book all on my own, but I couldn't. KJ's tireless work helping me think things through, listening to a thousand speech fragments, helping me find and format resources and citations, and quite literally keeping me alive during several months of involuntary bed rest, plus her effortless coolness, brilliance, and grace, are the only reasons you are holding this book in your hands. Our long little dog, Ume, watched me write well past sunrise every night for weeks in a row, and his contributions were invaluable.* I also need to thank the big man who gives me hope every Sunday: Aaron

---

*   I gave Ume a copy of the book to read. He told me it was "trash" and started eating it. Ume loves trash.

Rodgers, the greatest quarterback in the NFL. I would trade my every bone to give him what he needs to win four more rings, if that's what it took, and that's why I need single-payer healthcare.

Lastly, thank you for buying my book. That's awful nice of you.

ENDNOTES

INTRODUCTION

1. Associated Press. "Former Arkansas Lawmaker Charged in Scheme to Bribe Judge." *Times Record*, January 11, 2019. https://www.swtimes .com/news/20190111/former-arkansas-lawmaker-charged-in -scheme-to-bribe-judge. 28, 2019 Cheves, John. "He Writes Laws That Help Kentucky's Low-Rated Nursing Homes. He Also Works for Them." *Lexington Herald Leader*, September 27, 2018. https://www.kentucky.com/news/local/watchdog/article 217593015.html. Besson, Eric. "State Legislator Reveals Work Ties to Owner of Nursing Homes." *Arkansas Democrat Gazette*, January 27, 2019. www.arkansasonline.com/news/2019/jan/27/legislator-reveals -work-ties-to-owner-o/.
2. McGovern, Laura. "The Relative Contribution of Multiple Determinants to Health." *Health Affairs*, August 21, 2014. https://www .healthaffairs.org/do/10.1377/hpb20140821.404487/full/.

PART I: WHAT WE GOT

1. Sawyer, Bradley, and Cynthia Cox. "How Does Health Spending in the U.S. Compare to Other Countries?" *Peterson-Kaiser Health System Tracker* (blog). December 7, 2018. https://www.healthsystemtracker. org/chart-collection/health-spending-u-s-compare-countries/.

2. Anderson, Gerard. *Chronic Conditions: Making the Case for Ongoing Care*. Baltimore, MD: John Hopkins University, 2004.

3. Christopher, Andrea S., D.U. Himmelstein, Steffie Woolhandler, and Danny McCormick. "The Effects of Household Medical Expenditures on Income Inequality in the United States." *American Journal of Public Health*, 108(3), 351-354. doi: http://dx.doi.org.ezp-prod1.hul.harvard.edu/10.2105/AJPH.2017.304213. Newkirk II, Vann R. "The American Health-Care System Increases Income Inequality." *The Atlantic*, January 19, 2018. https://www.theatlantic.com/politics/archive/2018/01/health-care-income-inequality-premiums-deductibles-costs/550997/. ("In 2014, 9.28 million Americans whose incomes before their medical outlays were above poverty were pushed into near poverty (150% of FPL) when medical outlays were subtracted from their family incomes. Similarly, 7.013 million were lowered into poverty (below 100% of the FPL), and for 3.946 million, medical outlays reduced their incomes into the extreme poverty range (below 50% of the FPL)").

4. Claxton, Gary, Bradley Sawyer, and Nolan Sroczynski. "How Do Health Expenditures Vary across the Population?" *Peterson-Kaiser Health System Tracker* (blog), January 16, 2019. https://www.healthsystemtracker.org/chart-collection/health-expenditures-vary-across-population/#item-pocket-spending-health-services-almost-concentrated-overall-health-spending_2015 ("One percent of the popuation accounted for nearly a fifth of all out-of-pocket spending on health services in 2015, and the top 5% of spenders accounted for 45%. At the other end of the spectrum, the 50% of the population with the lowest out-of-pocket spending accounted for 2% of all out-of-pocket health spending.")

5. "Health Care Costs: A Primer." *The Henry J. Kaiser Family Foundation* (blog), May 12, 2012. https://www.kff.org/report-section/health-care-costs-a-primer-2012-report/.

6. Johnston, David W., Carol Propper, and Michael A. Shields. "Comparing Subjective and Objective Measures of Health: Evidence from Hypertension for the Income/Health Gradient." *Journal of Health Economics* 28, no. 3 (May 2009): 540–52. doi:10.1016/j.jhealeco.2009.02.010.

7.   Truven Health Analytics. "The Cost of Having a Baby in the United States: Executive Summary." Truven Health Analytics Marketscan Study, January 2013. http://transform.childbirthconnection.org /wp-content/uploads/2013/01/Cost-of-Having-a-Baby-Executive -Summary.pdf.

INSURANCE

8.   Kao, Helen, Rebecca Conant, Theresa Soriano, and Wayne Mc-Cormick. "The Past, Present, and Future of House Calls." *Clinics in Geriatric Medicine*, 25, no. 1 (February 2009): 19–34. ("House calls dropped from 40% of physician encounters in 1930 to 10% by 1950 and less than 1% by 1980.")

9.   Hoffman, Beatrix Rebecca. *Health Care for Some: Rights and Rationing in the United States Since 1930*. Chicago: University of Chicago Press, 2013.

10. Ross, Joseph H. "The Committee on the Costs of Medical Care and the History of Health Insurance in the United States," *Einstein Quarterly*, 19 (2002): 130. Ross cites M. Davis. "The American Approach to Health Insurance." *Milbank Memorial Fund Quarterly* 12 (1934): 211-215 as the source of these data.

11. Ibid. ("By 1929, hospital costs (not including doctors' and private nurses' hospital bills) were 13 percent of a total family medical bill.")

12. Blumberg, Alex, and Adam Davidson. "Accidents Of History Created U.S. Health System." NPR, October 22, 2009. https://www .npr.org/templates/story/story.php?storyId=114045132.

UNINSURANCE

13. Haefner, Morgan. "America's Uninsured Rate Climbs to 15.5%." Becker's Hospital Review, May 1, 2018. https://www.beckershospitalreview .com/payer-issues/america-s-uninsured-rate-climbs-to-15-5.html.

14. "Key Facts about the Uninsured Population." *The Henry J. Kaiser Family Foundation* (blog), December 7, 2018. https://www.kff.org /uninsured/fact-sheet/key-facts-about-the-uninsured-population/.

15. Institute of Medicine (US) Committee on the Consequences of Un-insurance. "Effects of Health Insurance on Health." In *Care Without Coverage: Too Little, Too Late*, 47. Washington DC: National Academies Press (US), 2002.

16. Cercere, David. "New Study Finds 45,000 Deaths Annually Linked to Lack of Health Coverage." *Harvard Gazette* (blog), September 17, 2009. https://news.harvard.edu/gazette/story/2009/09/new-study -finds-45000-deaths-annually-linked-to-lack-of-health-coverage/.

17. Collins, Sara R., Herman K. Bhupal, and Michelle M. Doty. "Health Insurance Coverage Eight Years After the ACA." Commonwealth Fund, February 7, 2019. https://www.commonwealthfund.org/publications /issue-briefs/2019/feb/health-insurance-coverage-eight-years-after-aca.

PUBLIC INSURANCE

18. The Boards of Trustees, Federal Hospital Insurance and Federal Supplementary Medical Insurance Trust Funds. "The 2018 Annual Report of the Boards of Trustees of the Federal Hospital Insurance and Federal Supplementary Medical Insurance Trust Funds." Center for Medicare and Medicaid Services, June 05, 2018. Accessed February 28, 2019. https://www.cms.gov/Research-Statis tics-Data-and-Systems/Statistics-Trends-and-Reports/Reports TrustFunds/downloads/tr2018.pdf.

19. Cross, Jory. "Plan Your Medicare Health Costs for Retirement." Medi-care.com, August 21, 2014. https://medicare.com/resources/plan -your-medicare-health-costs-for-retirement/.

20. Curto, Vilsa, Liran Einav, Amy Finkelstein, Jonathan Levin, and Jay Bhattacharya. "Healthcare Spending and Utilization in Public and Private Medicare." NBER Working Paper No. 23090, National Bureau of Economic Research, Cambridge, MA, January 2017. https://doi.org/10.3386/w23090.

21. Levinson, Daniel R. "Medicare Advantage Appeal Outcomes and Audit Findings Raise Concerns About Service and Payment Deni-als." U.S. Department of Health and Human Services Office of In-

spector General, September 2018. https://oig.hhs.gov/oei/reports/
oei-09-16-00410.pdf.

22. McGuire, Thomas G., Joseph P. Newhouse, and Anna D.
    Sinaiko. "An Economic History of Medicare Part C." *The Milbank
    Quarterly* 89, no. 2 (June 2011): 289–332. https://doi.org/10.1111
    /j.1468-0009.2011.00629.x.

23. Walsh, Mary Williams. "A Whistle-Blower Tells of Health Insurers
    Bilking Medicare." *New York Times*, May 15, 2017 https://www.ny
    times.com/2017/05/15/business/dealbook/a-whistle-blower-tells
    -of-health-insurers-bilking-medicare.html.

24. Paradise, Julia. "Data Note: A Large Majority of Physicians Partici-
    pate in Medicaid." *The Henry J. Kaiser Family Foundation* (blog), May 10,
    2017. https://www.kff.org/medicaid/issue-brief/data-note-a-large
    -majority-of-physicians-participate-in-medicaid/.

25. Coleman, Christopher E. "Trump Administratin's New Policay Al-
    lowing States to Deny Medicaid to Unemployed Workers Will Harm
    Tennessee Families." Tennessee Justice Center, January 26, 2018.
    https://www.tnjustice.org/wp-content/uploads/2018/01/Trump
    -Administrations-New-Policy-on-Unemployed-Workers.pdf. ("Ten-
    nCare has struggled to implement even basic changes to the Med-
    icaid eligibility and enrollment process required by the Affordable
    Care Act. Its new computerized eligibility system, the TennCare El-
    igibility Determination System (TEDS), is still not operational over
    four years after it was supposed to be completed [which] has created
    months-long delays in coverage [and] . . . caused numerous eligible
    individuals to be wrongfully terminated from the program.")

26. Garfield, Rachel, Robin Rudowitz, MaryBeth Musumeci,
    and Anthony Damico. "Implications of Work Requirements
    in Medicaid: What Does the Data Say?" *The Henry J. Kaiser
    Family Foundation* (blog), July 23, 2018. https://www.kff.org
    /medicaid/issue-brief/implications-of-work-requirements-in
    -medicaid-what-does-the-data-say/.

27. Bagalman, Erin. *The Number of Veterans That Use VA Health Care Ser-
    vices: A Fact Sheet.* Washington, D.C. Congressional Research Ser-

vice, June 3, 2014. https://fas.org/sgp/crs/misc/R43579.pdf.

28. Vanden Heuvel, Katrina. "Why Is the VA Suffering From a Lack of Resources in the First Place?" *The Nation*, June 29, 2015. https://www.thenation.com/article/why-va-suffering-lack-resources-first-place/.

29. Clason, Lauren. "Senators Back Agent Orange Benefits. The VA Is Not Convinced." *Roll Call*, August 2, 2018. https://www.rollcall.com/news/politics/senate-agent-orange-veterans-affairs.

30. Devine, Curt. "307,000 Vets May Have Died Awaiting VA Care, Report Says." CNN, September 3, 2015. https://www.cnn.com/2015/09/02/politics/va-inspector-general-report/index.html.

PRIVATE INSURANCE

31. Barnett, Jessica C., Edward R. Berchick, and Emily Hood. "Health Insurance Coverage in the United States: 2017." United States Census Bureau, September 12, 2018. https://www.census.gov/library/publications/2018/demo/p60-264.html. ("In 2017, private health insurance coverage continued to be more prevalent than government coverage, at 67.2 percent and 37.7 percent, respectively.")

32. Schoen, Cathy, and Sara R. Collins. "The Big Five Health Insurers' Membership And Revenue Trends: Implications For Public Policy." *Health Affairs* 36, no. 12 (December 2017): 2185–94. https://doi.org/10.1377/hlthaff.2017.0858.

33. Heitz, David. "Insurers Accused of Keeping HIV Medications Out of Patients' Reach." *Healthline*, May 30, 2014. https://www.healthline.com/health-news/lawsuit-accuses-insurers-withholding-hiv-medication-053014.

34. Kennedy, Patrick J. "Why We Must End Insurance Discrimination against Mental Health Care." *Harvard Journal on Legislation* 41, no.2 (2004): 363–75.

COST

35. Claxton, Gary, Matthew Rae, Larry Levitt, and Cynthia Cox. "How Have Healthcare Prices Grown in the U.S. Over Time?"

Peterson-Kaiser Health System Tracker (blog), May 8, 2018.https:// www.healthsystemtracker.org/chart-collection/how-have-health care-prices-grown-in-the-u-s-over-time; Anderson, Gerard F., Uwe E. Reinhardt, Peter S. Hussey, and Varduhi Petrosyan. "It's The Prices, Stupid: Why The United States Is So Different From Other Countries." *Health Affairs* 22, no. 3 (May 2003): 89–105. https://doi. org/10.1377/hlthaff.22.3.89.Anderson, Gerard F., Peter Hussey, and Varduhi Petrosyan. "It's Still The Prices, Stupid: Why The US Spends So Much On Health Care, And A Tribute To Uwe Reinhardt." *Health Affairs* 38, no. 1 (January 2019): 87–95. https://doi .org/10.1377/hlthaff.2018.05144.

36. Papanicolas, Irene, Liana R. Woskie, and Ashish K. Jha. "Health Care Spending in the United States and Other High-Income Countries." Abstract.*JAMA* 319, no. 10 (March 13, 2018): 1024. https://doi.org/10.1001 /jama.2018.1150. ("On key measures of health care resources per capita (hospital beds, physicians, and nurses), the US still provides significantly fewer resources compared to the OECD median country. Since the US is not consuming greater resources than other countries, the most logical factor is the higher prices paid in the US.")

37. *2018 Comparative Price Report: Variation in Medical and Hospital Prices by Country.* London. International Federation of Health Plans, May 2018.

38. Kliff, Sarah. "How Much Does an MRI Cost? In D.C., Anywhere from $400 to $1,861." *Washington Post*, March 13, 2013. https://www .washingtonpost.com/news/wonk/wp/2013/03/13/how-much -does-an-mri-cost-in-d-c-anywhere-from-400-to-1861.

39. Cooper, Zack, Stuart Craig, Martin Gaynor, and John Van Reenen. *The Price Ain't Right? Hospital Prices and Health Spending on the Privately Insured.* New Haven: Health Care Pricing Project, May 2015. https:// healthcarepricingproject.org/papers/paper-1.

40. Enriquez, Jof. "FDA's PMA Approval Rate Soars To 15-Year High." *Med Device Online* (blog), December 2, 2015. https://www.meddevice online.com/doc/fda-s-pma-approval-rate-soars-to-year-high-0001.

41. Rosenthal, Elisabeth. *An American Sickness: How Healthcare Became Big Business and How You Can Take It Back.* New York: Penguin Books, 2018.

42. Pollack, Andrew. "Drug Goes From $13.50 a Tablet to $750, Overnight." *New York Times*, September 20, 2015, https://www.nytimes.com/2015/09/21/business/a-huge-overnight-increase-in-a-drugs-price-raises-protests.html.

43. Luthra, Shefali. "'Pharma Bro' Shkreli Is In Prison, But Daraprim's Price Is Still High." *Kaiser Health News* (blog), May 4, 2018. https://khn.org/news/for-shame-pharma-bro-shkreli-is-in-prison-but-daraprims-price-is-still-high/.

44. Swetlitz, Ike. "High Price of EpiPen Spurs Consumers, EMTs To Resort to Syringes for Allergic Reactions." *STAT News*. February 12, 2018. https://www.statnews.com/2016/07/06/epipen-prices-allergies/.

45. Cha, Ariana Eunjung. "Senator's Daughter Who Raised Price of EpiPen Got Paid $19 Million Salary, Perks in 2015." *Washington Post*, August 24, 2016. https://www.washingtonpost.com/news/to-your-health/wp/2016/08/24/senators-daughter-who-raised-price-of-epipen-got-paid-19-million-salary-perks-in-2015/.

46. Hua Xinyang, Natalie Carvalho, Michelle Tew, Elbert S. Huang, William H. Herman, Philip Clarke. "Expenditures and Prices of Antihyperglycemic Medications in the United States: 2002–2013." *JAMA* 315, no. 13 (April 5, 2016): 1400–1402. doi:10.1001/jama.2016.0126.

47. Herkert, Darby M., Pavithra Vijayakumar, Jing Luo, Jeremy Schwartz, Tracy L. Rabin, Eunice M. Defilippo, and Kasia J. Lipska. "Cost-Related Insulin Underuse Is Common and Associated with Poor Glycemic Control." Supplement, *Diabetes* 67, no. 1 (July 1, 2018): 2–OR. https://doi.org/10.2337/db18-2-OR.

48. Ramsey, Lydia. "There's Something Odd about the Way Insulin Prices Change." *Business Insider*, September 17, 2016. https://www.businessinsider.com/rising-insulin-prices-track-competitors-closely-2016-9.

49. Hagan, Allison. "Protesters at Sanofi in Cambridge Decry High Price of Insulin." *Boston Globe*, November 16, 2018. https://www.bostonglobe.com/business/2018/11/16/protesters-sanofi-cambridge-decry-high-price-of-insulin/MeEajamQHARWqDTQKXqPVL/story.html.

50. Goldman, Dana P., Geoffrey Joyce, Rocio Ribero, and Karen Van

Nuys. "Overpaying for Prescription Drugs: The Copay Clawback Phenomenon." USC Leonard D. Schaffer Center for Health Policy & Economics, March 12, 2018, https://healthpolicy.usc.edu/wp-content/uploads/2018/03/2018.03_Overpaying20for20Prescription20 Drugs_White20Paper_v.1-2.pdf/.

51. Ibid.

52. Yost, David. *Ohio Department of Medicaid Report on MCP Pharmacy Benefit Manager Performance*. Columbus: The Office of the Auditor of the State of Ohio, August 16, 2018. https://ohioauditor.gov/auditsearch/Reports/2018/Medicaid_Pharmacy_Services_2018_Franklin.pdf.

53. Thomas, Katie. "Meet the Rebate, the New Villain of High Drug Prices." *The New York Times*, July 27, 2018. https://www.nytimes.com/2018/07/27/health/rebates-high-drug-prices-trump.html.

54. Kodjak, Alison. "Hepatitis Drug Among The Most Costly For Medicaid." NPR, December 15, 2015. https://www.npr.org/sections/health-shots/2015/12/15/459873815/hepatitis-drug-among-the-most-costly-for-medicaid.

55. Gokhale, Ketaki. "The Same Pill That Costs $1,000 in the U.S. Sells for $4 in India." *Chicago Tribune*, January 4, 2016. https://www.chicagotribune.com/business/ct-drug-price-sofosbuvir-sovaldi-india-us-20160104-story.html.

56. Aleccia, JoNel. "Judge Orders Washington Medicaid to Provide Lifesaving Hepatitis C Drugs for All." *Seattle Times*, May 28, 2016. https://www.seattletimes.com/seattle-news/health/judge-orders-apple-health-to-cover-hepatitis-c-drugs-for-all/.

57. Kopp, Emily. "Groups That Represent Patients Are Ranking in Donations from Big Pharma." *Money*, March 2, 2017. http://money.com/money/4688501/patient-advocacy-groups-donations-from-pharma/.

58. Trickey, Erick. "A Palace Away From Home." *Cleveland Magazine*, January 1, 2003. https://clevelandmagazine.com/in-the-cle/people/articles/a-palace-away-from-home.

59. Diamond, Dan. "How the Cleveland Clinic Grows Healthier While its Neighbors Stay Sick." *POLITICO*, July 17, 2017. http://www.politico.com/interactives/2017/obamacare-cleveland-clinic-non-profit-hospital-taxes/.

60. Ibid.

61. Twedt, Steve. "UPMC Maintains It Has No Employees." *Pittsburgh Post-Gazette*. Nov. 11, 2013. https://www.post-gazette.com/business /2013/11/12/UPMC-maintains-it-has-no-employees/stories/2013 11120158.

62. Osdol, Paul Van. "Big Water Customers Owe Millions in Delinquent Bills." WTAE, November 5, 2015. https://www.wtae.com/article /big-water-customers-owe-millions-in-delinquent-bills/7474920.

63. Deitch, Charlie. "UPMC Opens Food Bank for Struggling Employees, Misses Point Completely (UPDATED)." *Pittsburgh City Paper Blogh* (blog), December 11, 2012. https://www.pgh citypaper.com/Blogh/archives/2012/12/11/upmc-opens-food-bank -for-struggling-employees-misses-point-completely.

64. Cooper, Zack, Stuart Craig, Martin Gaynor, Nir J. Harish, Harlan M. Krumholz, and John Van Reenen. "Hospital Prices Grew Substantially Faster Than Physician Prices For Hospital-Based Care In 2007–14." *Health Affairs* 38, no. 2 (2019): 184-89. https://doi.org /10.1377/hlthaff.2018.05424.

65. Koechlini, Francette, Paul Konijnii, Luca Lorenzonii, and Paul Schreyeri. "Comparing Hospital and Health Prices and Volumes Internationally: Results of a Eurostat/OECD Project." OECD Health Working Papers no. 75, Organisation for Economic Co-operation, Maris, August 26, 2014. https://doi.org/10.1787 /5jxznwrj32mp-en.

66. Rabin, Roni Caryn. "Appendectomy Can Cost $1,500—or $182,955." *Seattle Times*, April 23, 2012. https://www.seattletimes.com/nation -world/appendectomy-can-cost-1500-8212-or-182955/.

67. Smith, Jacquelyn. "The Best- And Worst-Paying Jobs For Doctors." *Forbes*, July 20, 2012. https://www.forbes.com/sites/jacquelyn smith/2012/07/20/the-best-and-worst-paying-jobs-for-doctors-2/.

68. Rabin, Roni Caryn. "15-Minute Visits Take A Toll On The Doctor-Patient Relationship." *Kaiser Health News* (blog), April 21, 2014. https://khn.org/news/15-minute-doctor-visits/.

69. Ofri, Danielle. "The Patients vs. Paperwork Problem for Doctors." *The New York Times*, November 14, 2017. https://www.nytimes

.com/2017/11/14/well/live/the-patients-vs-paperwork-problem-for
-doctors.html.

70. "Professionally Active Physicians." *The Henry J. Kaiser Family Foundation* (blog), October 17, 2018. https://www.kff.org/other/state-indicator/total-active-physicians/.

71. Council on Graduate Medical Education. "Summary of Eighth Report." Health Resources & Services Administration, November 1996. https://www.hrsa.gov/advisorycommittees/bhpradvisory/cogme/Reports/eighthreport.html.

72. Wennberg, John E. 2010. *Tracking Medicine: A Researcher's Quest to Understand Health Care.* New York: Oxford University Press, 2010.

73. "2018 M&A In Review: The Year in Numbers." Kaufman Hall. Accessed February 28, 2019. https://mnareview.kaufmanhall.com/the-year-in-numbers.

74. Capps, Cory, David Dranove, and Christopher Ody. "The Effect of Hospital Acquisitions of Physician Practices on Prices and Spending." *Journal of Health Economics* 59 (May 2018): 139–52. https://doi.org/10.1016/j.jhealeco.2018.04.001.

"SKIN IN THE GAME": PUNISHING PEOPLE FOR GETTING SICK

75. Brook, Robert H., Emmett B. Keeler, Kathleen N. Lohr, Joseph P. Newhouse, John E. Ware, William H. Rogers, Allyson Ross Davies, Cathy D. Sherbourne, George A. Goldberg, Patricia Camp, Caren Kamberg, Arleen Leibowitz, Joan Keesey, and David Reboussin. *The Health Insurance Experiment: A Classic RAND Study Speaks to the Current Health Care Reform Debate.* Santa Monica, CA: RAND Corporation, 2006. https://www.rand.org/pubs/research_briefs/RB9174.html.

76. *2017 Employer Health Benefits Survey—Section 8: High-Deductible Health Plans with Savings Option.* The Henry J. Kaiser Family Foundation, San Francisco, September 19, 2017. https://www.kff.org/report-section/ehbs-2017-section-8-high-deductible-health-plans-with-savings-option/.

77. *Report on the Economic Well-Being of U.S. Households in 2017.* Board of Governors of the Federal Reserve System: Washington, D.C., May 2018. https://www.federalreserve.gov/publications/files/2017-report-economic-well-being-us-households-201805.pdf.

78. Kenen, Joanne. "Looking at the Conservative 'Heritage' of Some Core ACA Features." *Association of Health Care Journalists* (blog), February 28, 2017. https://healthjournalism.org/blog/2017/02/looking-at-the-conservative-heritage-of-some-core-aca-features/.

79. "Key Facts about the Uninsured Population." *The Henry J. Kaiser Family Foundation* (blog), December 7, 2018. https://www.kff.org/uninsured/fact-sheet/key-facts-about-the-uninsured-population/.

80. *Overview of the Uninsured in the United States: A Summary of the 2011 Current Population Survey.* Office of the Assistant Secretary for Planning and Evaluation, Department of Health and Human Services: Washington, D.C., June 13, 2015. https://aspe.hhs.gov/basic-report/overview-uninsured-united-states-summary-2011-current-population-survey.

81. "Key Facts about the Uninsured Population." *The Henry J. Kaiser Family Foundation* (blog).

82. "Medicaid Expansion Enrollment." *The Henry J. Kaiser Family Foundation* (blog), December 19, 2018. https://www.kff.org/health-reform/state-indicator/medicaid-expansion-enrollment/.

83. Bloomberg. "Since Obamacare Became Law, 20 Million More Americans Have Gained Health Insurance." *Fortune.* November 15, 2018. http://fortune.com/2018/11/15/obamacare-americans-with-health-insurance-uninsured/.

84. fat guy from dynasty warriors (@crushingbort). "hmm well I'd say I'm fiscally conservative but socially very liberal. the problems are bad but their causes . . . their causes are very good." Twitter. May 5, 2015, 2:44 a.m. Tweet deleted.

85. Sommers, Benjamin D., Katherine Baicker, and Arnold M. Epstein. "Mortality and Access to Care among Adults after State Medicaid Expansions." *New England Journal of Medicine 367*, no. 11 (September 13, 2012): 1025–34. https://doi.org/10.1056/NEJMsa1202099.

THE MOST DANGEROUS PLACE

86. "New Study: U.S. Ranks Last Among High-Income Nations on Preventable Deaths, Lagging Behind as Others Improve More Rapidly." Commonwealth Fund, September 23, 2011. https://www.commonwealthfund.org/press-release/2011/new-study-us-ranks-last-among-high-income-nations-preventable-deaths-lagging/.

87. Villarosa, Linda. "Why America's Black Mothers and Babies Are in a Life-or-Death Crisis." *New York Times Magaine*, April 11, 2018. https://www.nytimes.com/2018/04/11/magazine/black-mothers-babies-death-maternal-mortality.html.

88. Martin, Nina. "The Last Person You'd Expect to Die in Childbirth." *ProPublica*, May 12, 2017. https://www.propublica.org/article/die-in-childbirth-maternal-death-rate-health-care-system.

89. Borchelt, Gretchen. "The Impact Poverty Has on Women's Health." American Bar Association. Accessed May 26, 2019. https://www.americanbar.org/groups/crsj/publications/human_rights_magazine_home/the-state-of-healthcare-in-the-united-states/poverty-on-womens-health/.

90. Hobbes, Michael. "Why Did AIDS Ravage the U.S. More Than Any Other Developed Country?" *New Republic*, May 12, 2014. https://newrepublic.com/article/117691/aids-hit-united-states-harder-other-developed-countries-why. ("AIDS has claimed more lives in NYC than in Spain, Italy, the Netherlands and Switzerland combined.")

91. Osborn, Robin, Michelle M. Doty, Donald Moulds, Dana O. Sarnak, and Arnav Shah. "Older Americans Were Sicker And Faced More Financial Barriers To Health Care Than Counterparts In Other Countries." *Health Affairs* 36, no. 12 (December 2017): 2123–32. https://doi.org/10.1377/hlthaff.2017.1048.

92. Kochanek, Kenneth D., Sherry L. Murphy, Jiaquan Xu, and Elizabeth Arias. *Mortality in the United States*, 2016. NCHS Data Brief: Washington D.C., December 2017. https://www.cdc.gov/nchs/data/databriefs/db293.pdf.

93. Ibid.

PART II: WHAT WE WANT

WHAT IS SINGLE-PAYER?

1. Face (@Arr). "Being a human rules because we're big shitty malfunctioning robots made out of this gross goo technology that we baaaaarely understand." Twitter. February 29, 2012, 10:58 a.m. https://twitter.com/Arr/status/174931480693325824.

2. Wallace, Jacob, and Zirui Song. "Traditional Medicare Versus Private Insurance: How Spending, Volume, And Price Change At Age Sixty-Five." *Health Affairs* 35, no. 5 (May 1, 2016): 864–72. https://doi.org/10.1377/hlthaff.2015.1195.

3. "NHE-Fact-Sheet," Centers for Medicaid and Medicare Services. Accessed February 20, 2019. https://www.cms.gov/research-statistics -data-and-systems/statistics-trends-and-reports/nationalhealth expendata/nhe-fact-sheet.html.

4. Himmelstein, David U. and Steffie Woolhandler. "The Current and Projected Taxpayer Shares of US Health Costs." *American Journal of Public Health* 106, no. 3 (March 1, 2016): pp. 449-452. https://www .ncbi.nlm.nih.gov/pmc/articles/PMC4880216/.

5. Blahous, Charles. *The Costs of a National Single-Payer Healthcare System*. Arlington, VA: Mercatus Working Paper, July 2018. https://www.mercatus.org/system/files/blahous-costs-medicare -mercatus-working-paper-v1_1.pdf

6. Pollin, Robert, James Heintz, Peter Arno, Jeannette Wicks-Lim, and Michael Ash. "Economic Analysis of Medicare for All." Political Economy Research Institute, November 30, 2018. https:// www.peri.umass.edu/publication/item/1127-economic-analysis -of-medicare-for-all.

7. "Medicare for All: Leaving No One Behind." BernieSanders.com. Accessed May 26, 2019. https://web.archive.org/web/20190214082511/ https://berniesanders.com/issues/medicare-for-all/ ("Under this plan, a family of four earning $50,000 would pay just $466 per year to the single-payer program, amounting to a savings of over $5,800 for that family each year.")

8. "National Health Expenditure Projections 2018-2027." Centers for Medicare & Medicaid Services. Accessed May 26, 2019. https://www.cms.gov/Research-Statistics-Data-and-Systems/Statistics-Trends-and-Reports/NationalHealthExpendData/Downloads/ForecastSummary.pdf.

9. Reeves, Aaron, Sanjay Basu, Martin McKee, Christopher Meissner, and David Stuckler. "Does investment in the health sector promote or inhibit economic growth?" *Globalization and Health* 9 (September 23, 2013): 43. https://doi.org/10.1186/1744-8603-9-43.

10. Cox, Cynthia, and Bradley Sawyer. "How does health spending in the U.S. compare to other countries?" *Peterson-Kaiser Health System Tracker* (blog), December 7, 2018. https://www.healthsystemtracker.org/chart-collection/health-spending-u-s-compare-countries/.

11. Coombs, Bertha. "As Obamacare twists in political winds, top insurers made $6 billion (not that there is anything wrong with that)" CNBC. August 5, 2017. https://www.cnbc.com/2017/08/05/top-health-insurers-profit-surge-29-percent-to-6-billion-dollars.html.

12. "Health at a Glance 2017: OECD Indicators." OECD. Accessed May 26, 2019. https://www.oecd.org/unitedstates/Health-at-a-Glance-2017-Key-Findings-UNITED-STATES.pdf.

13. Holahan, John, Matthew Buettgens, Lisa Clemans-Cope, Melissa M. Favreault, Linda J. Blumberg, and Siyabonga Ndwandwe. "The Sanders Single-Payer Health Care Plan: The Effect on National Health Expenditures and Federal and Private Spending." Urban Institute, May 9, 2016. https://www.urban.org/research/publication/sanders-single-payer-health-care-plan-effect-national-health-expenditures-and-federal-and-private-spending/view/full_report. ("Private health care spending by households and employers would drop as the federal government would absorb their spending under current law. Private sector expenditures for these groups would decrease by $1.7 trillion in 2017 and by $21.9 trillion between 2017 and 2026. These considerable savings would partially offset the impact on the private sector of new taxes required to pay for the Sanders plan.")

14. Barber, Sarah L., Ankit Kumar, Tomas Roubal, Francesca Colombo, and Luca Lorenzoni. "Harnessing the private health sector

by using prices as a policy instrument: Lessons learned from South Africa." *Health Policy* 122, no. 5 (May 2018): 558–64. https://doi.org /10.1016/j.healthpol.2018.03.018.

15. Boehler, Adam, and Mary Mayhew. "Strong Start for Mothers and Newborns." Department of Health and Human Services (memo), November 9, 2018. https://www.medicaid.gov/federal-policy-guidance /downloads/cib110918.pdf.

16. "Medicaid Redesign Team Supportive Housing Initiative." Accessed February 28, 2019. Evaluation. New York State Department of Health, September 2017. https://www.health.ny.gov/health_care /medicaid/redesign/supportive_housing_initiatives.htm.

17. Diaz-Alvarez, Enrique. "The Backroom Deal That Could've Given Us Single-Payer." *Jacobin*, December 9, 2013. http://jacobinmag .com/2013/12/the-backroom-deal-that-couldve-led-to-single-payer/.

18. Bruenig, Matt. "Single Payer Myths: Redundant Health Administration Workers." People's Policy Project, September 19, 2017. https://www.peoplespolicyproject.org/2017/09/19/single-payer -myths-redundant-health-administration-workers/.

19. Majeed, Azeem, Dominique Allwood, Kim Foley, and Andrew Bindman. "Healthcare Outcomes and Quality in the NHS: How Do We Compare and How Might the NHS Improve?" *BMJ* 362 (July 13, 2018): k3036. https://doi.org/10.1136/bmj.k3036.

WHAT ISN'T SINGLE-PAYER?

20. Keller, Megan. "Seventy Percent of Americans Support 'Medicare for All' in New Poll." *The Hill*, August 23, 2018. https://thehill.com /policy/healthcare/403248-poll-seventy-percent-of-americans -support-medicare-for-all.

21. Faust, Timothy. "The Very Bad Politics of 'Putting Healthcare Over Politics.'" *Splinter*, February 8, 2018. https://splinternews.com/the -very-bad-politics-of-putting-healthcare-over-politi-1822806820.

22. Grim, Ryan. "Top Nancy Pelosi Aide Privately Tells Insurance Executives Not to Worry About Democrats Pushing 'Medi-

care for All.'" *The Intercept*, February 5, 2019. https://theintercept
.com/2019/02/05/nancy-pelosi-medicare-for-all/.

23. Jacobson, Gretchen, Anthony Damico, and Tricia Neuman. "Medicare Advantage 2019 Spotlight: First Look." *The Henry J. Kaiser Family
Foundation* (blog), October 16, 2018. https://www.kff.org/medicare
/issue-brief/medicare-advantage-2019-spotlight-first-look/.

24. Dinerstein, Chuck. "The Department of Justice Believes United
Healthcare Is Defrauding Medicare." American Council on
Science and Health, February 21, 2017. https://www.acsh.org
/news/2017/02/21/department-justice-believes-united-healthcare
-defrauding-medicare-10885.

25. Walsh, Mary Williams. "UnitedHealth Overbilled Medicare
by Billions, U.S. Says in Suit." *The New York Times*, May 19, 2017.
https://www.nytimes.com/2017/05/19/business/dealbook/united
health-sued-medicare-overbilling.html.

26. "One of Nation's Largest Dialysis Providers Agrees To $270M
Settlement over Medicare Advantage Fraud." *Kaiser Health News*
(blog), October 2, 2018. https://khn.org/morning-breakout/one-of
-nations-largest-dialysis-providers-agrees-to-270m-settlement
-over-medicare-advantage-fraud/.

27. The CAP Health Policy Team. "Medicare Extra for All." Center
for American Progress, February 22, 2018. https://www.american
progress.org/issues/healthcare/reports/2018/02/22/447095/medi
care-extra-for-all/.

28. Grim, Ryan. "Top Nancy Pelosi Aide Privately Tells Insurance Executives Not to Worry About Democrats Pushing 'Medicare for All.'"

29. Ginneken, Ewout van, Katherine Swartz, and Philip Van der Wees.
"Health Insurance Exchanges In Switzerland And The Netherlands
Offer Five Key Lessons For The Operations Of US Exchanges."
Health Affairs 32, no. 4 (April 1, 2013): 744–52. https://doi.org/10.1377/
hlthaff.2012.0948.

30. Riley, Wayne J. "Health Disparities: Gaps in Access, Quality and Affordability of Medical Care." *Transactions of the American Clinical and Climatological Association* 123 (2012): 167–74; Jha, Ashish K., E. John Orav, and Arnold M. Epstein. "Low-Quality, High-Cost Hospitals, Mainly in South, Care for Sharply Higher Shares of Elderly Black, Hispanic, and Medicaid Patients." *Health Affairs* 30, no. 10 (October 2011): 1904–11. https://doi.org/10.1377/hlthaff.2011.0027.

31. "97 Rural Hospital Closures: January 2010–Present." Sheps Center. Accessed February 28, 2019. https://www.shepscenter.unc.edu/programs -projects/rural-health/rural-hospital-closures/. Updated regularly.

32. Kliff, Sarah. "How Obamacare Saved Detroit." *Vox*, July 25, 2017. https://www.vox.com/policy-and-politics/2017/7/25/16001508 /obamacare-detroit-medicaid-repeal. (CHASS is a great example of what a healthcare center can do.)

33. "Home Health Aides and Personal Care Aides." *In Occupational Outlook Handbook*. U.S. Bureau of Labor Statistics, Accessed February 28, 2019. https://www.bls.gov/ooh/healthcare/home-health-aides-and-personal-care-aides.htm#tab-6. Updated April 12, 2019.

34. Brown, Leanna. *Good and Cheap: Eating Well on $4/Day*. Self-published, www.leannebrown.com, Version 1.1, August 2014. https:// cookbooks.leannebrown.com/good-and-cheap.pdf.

35. Brooker, S., A.C. Clements, P.J. Hotez, S.I. Hay, A.J. Tatem, D.A. Bundy, and R.W. Snow. "The Co-Distribution of Plasmodium Falciparum and Hookworm among African Schoolchildren." *Malaria Journal* 5 (2006): 99. https://www.ncbi.nlm.nih.gov/pubmed /17083720.

36. McKenna, Megan L., Shannon McAtee, Patricia E. Bryan, Rebecca Jeun, Tabitha Ward, Jacob Kraus, Maria E. Bottazzi, Peter J. Hotez, Catherine C. Flowers, and Rojelio Mejia. "Human Intestinal Parasite Burden and Poor Sanitation in Rural Alabama." *The American Journal of Tropical Medicine and Hygiene* 97, no. 5 (November 8, 2017): 1623–28. https://doi.org/10.4269/ajtmh.17-0396. http://www.ajtmh .org/content/journals/10.4269/ajtmh.17-0396.

37. Fehr, Rachel. "Insurer Participation on ACA Marketplaces, 2014–2019." *The Henry J. Kaiser Family Foundation (blog)*, November 14, 2018. https://www.kff.org/health-reform/issue-brief/insurer-participation-on-aca-marketplaces-2014-2019/.

38. "97 Rural Hospital Closures: January 2010–Present."

PART III: WHAT LIES BEYOND

1.   McGovern, Laura. "The Relative Contribution of Multiple Determinants to Health." *Health Affairs*, August 21, 2014. https://www.healthaffairs.org/do/10.1377/hpb20140821.404487/full/.

SOCIAL DETERMINANTS OF HEALTH

2. O'Connell, James J. *Premature Mortality in Homeless Populations: A Review of the Literature.* Nashville: National Health Care for the Homeless Council, December 2005. http://sbdww.org/wp-content/uploads/2011/04/PrematureMortalityFinal.pdf; Wright, J.D. "Poor People, Poor Health: The Health Status of the Homeless." In *Under the Safety Net: The Health and Social Welfare of the Homeless in the United States*, edited by Philip Brickner, Linda keen Scharer, and Barbara A. Conanan. New York: WW Norton & Co., 1990

3. "Medicaid and Supportive Housing." Supportive Housing Network of NY. Accessed February 28, 2019. https://shnny.org/budget-policy/state/medicaid-redesign/.

4. "Medicaid Redesign Team Supportive Housing Initiative." Accessed February 28, 2019. https://www.health.ny.gov/health_care/medicaid/redesign/supportive_housing_initiatives.htm. Updated April 2019.

5. Elejalde-Ruiz, Alexia. "Saving Lives, Saving Money: Hospitals Set Up Homeless Patients with Permanent Housing." *Chicago Tribune*, January 12, 2018. Accessed February 28, 2019. https://www.chicagotribune.com/business/ct-biz-hospitals-house-homeless-0114-story.html.

6. Gundersen, Craig, and James P. Ziliak. "Food Insecurity And Health Outcomes." *Health Affairs* 34, no. 11 (November 2015): 1830–39. https://doi.org/10.1377/hlthaff.2015.0645.

7. Ibid.

8. Ibid.

9. Ziliak, J.P., Craig Gundersen, and Margaret Haist. *The Causes, Consequences, and Future of Senior Hunger in America.* University of Kentucky, Center for Poverty Research: April 2008. https://pdfs.semantic scholar.org/8b96/75cf8502c5830aa48bfe59e3c3d4a3c99245.pdf.

10. Nathan, David M. "Long-Term Complications of Diabetes Mellitus." *New England Journal of Medicine* 328, no. 23 (June 10, 1993): 1676–85. https://doi.org/10.1056/NEJM199306103282306.

11. Dubowitz, Tamara, Madhumita Ghosh-Dastidar, Deborah A. Cohen, Robin Beckman, Elizabeth D. Steiner, Gerald P. Hunter, Karen R. Flórez, Christina Huang, Christine A. Vaughan, Jennifer C. Sloan, Shannon N. Zenk, Steven Cummins, and Rebecca L. Collins. "Diet and Perceptions Change with Supermarket introduction in a Food Desert, but Not Because of Supermarket Use." *Health Affairs* 34, no. 11 (November 2015): 1858–68. https://doi.org/10.1377/hlthaff.2015.0667.

12. Krukowski Rebecca A., Delia Smith West, Jean Harvey-Berino, T. Elaine Prewitt. "Neighborhood Impact on Healthy Food Availability and Pricing in Food Stores." *J Community Health* 35 no. 3 (June 2010): 315–320. https://www.ncbi.nlm.nih.gov/pmc/articles/PMC3071013. *J Community Health.* 2010;35(3):315-20t.

13. "Lead Poisoning and Health." World Health Organization. August 23, 2018. https://www.who.int/news-room/fact-sheets/detail/lead-poisoning-and-health.

14. Spicuzza, Mary, and Daniel Bice. "Protecting Milwaukee's Children: What We Know About the Latest Problems with the City's Lead Poisoning Prevention Efforts." *Milwaukee Journal Sentinel*, May 31, 2018. https://www.jsonline.com/story/news/politics/2018/05/31/city-milwaukee-faces-problems-programs-lead-poisoned-kids/658027002/.

15. Hahn, Robert A., and Benedict I. Truman. "Education Improves

Public Health and Promotes Health Equity." *International Journal of Health Services*, Evaluation 45, no. 4 (2015): 657–78. https://doi.org/10.1177/0020731415585986.

16. Center on Social Disparities in Health at University of California, San Francisco. "Gaps in Infant Mortality: How Do States Compare?" Prepared for the Robert Wood Johnson Foundation Commission to Build a Healthier America: 2008. http://www.commissiononhealth.org/PDF/tab6_78.pdf.

17. Cleland, J. G., and J. K. Van Ginneken. "Maternal Education and Child Survival in Developing Countries: The Search for Pathways of Influence." *Social Science & Medicine* 27, no. 12 (1988): 1357–68. https://www.ncbi.nlm.nih.gov/pubmed/3070762.

18. Reynolds, A. J., J. A. Temple, S. R. Ou, D. L. Robertson, J. P. Mersky, J. W. Topitzes, and M. D. Niles. "Effects Of A School-Based, Early Childhood Intervention on Adult Health and Well-Being: a 19-year Follow-Up of Low-Income Families." *Arch Pediatr Adolesc Med.* 161 no. 8 (2007): 730–739. https://www.ncbi.nlm.nih.gov/pubmed/17679653.

19. Marmot, Michael. "The Influence Of Income On Health: Views Of An Epidemiologist." *Health Affairs* 21, no. 2 (March 1, 2002): 31–46. https://doi.org/10.1377/hlthaff.21.2.31.

20. Komro, Kelli A., Melvin D. Livingston, Sara Markowitz, and Alexander C. Wagenaar. "The Effect of an Increased Minimum Wage on Infant Mortality and Birth Weight." *American Journal of Public Health* 106, no. 8 (August 1, 2016): 1514–1516 https://ajph.aphapublications.org/doi/10.2105/AJPH.2016.303268.

21. McLean, Katherine. "'There's Nothing Here': Deindustrialization as risk environment for overdose." *International Journal of Drug Policy* 29 (March 1, 2016): 19–26. https://doi.org/10.1016/j.drugpo.2016.01.009.

HOUSTON JAILS AS WAREHOUSES FOR THE SICK

22. Rayasam, Renuka. "Houston's Biggest Jail Wants to Shed Its Reputation as a Mental Health Treatment Center." *POLITICO*, July 9, 2018. Accessed February 28, 2019. https://politi.co/2JwHYAd.

23. Ford, Matt. "America's Largest Mental Hospital Is a Jail." *The Atlantic*, June 8, 2015. https://www.theatlantic.com/politics/archive/2015/06/americas-largest-mental-hospital-is-a-jail/395012/.

24. Bridges, Khiara M. *The Poverty of Privacy Rights*. Stanford: Stanford University Press, 2017.

25. I don't know how to cite this one. It's from a talk she gave and a friend then told me about. So I guess follow her on Twitter? @prisonculture

STRUCTURAL DETERMINANTS OF HEALTH RACISM

26. "Infant Mortality." Centers for Disease Control and Prevention. https://www.cdc.gov/reproductivehealth/maternalinfant health/infantmortality.htm. Updated March 2019.

27. Xu, Jiaquan, Sherry L. Murphy, Kenneth D. Kochanek, Brigham Bastian, and Elizabeth Arias. "Deaths: Final Data for 2016" *National Vital Statistics Reports* 67, no. 05 (July 6, 2018). https://www.cdc.gov/nchs/data/nvsr/nvsr67/nvsr67_05.pdf.

28. Curtin, P. D. "The Slavery Hypothesis for Hypertension among African Americans: The Historical Evidence." *American Journal of Public Health* 82, no. 12 (December 1992): 1681–86. https://www.ncbi.nlm.nih.gov/pmc/articles/PMC1694537/.

29. Hamilton, Erin, Jodi Berger Cardoso, Robert A. Hummer, and Yolanda C. Padilla. "Assimilation and Emerging Health Disparities among New Generations of U.S. Children." *Demographic Research* 25, no. 25 (December 8, 2011): 783–818. https://doi.org/10.4054/DemRes.2011.25.25.

30. Gee, Gilbert C., and Chandra L. Ford. "Structural Racism And Health Inequities: Old Issues, New Directions." Special issue, *Du Bois Review: Racial Inequality and Health* 8, no. 1 (Spring 2011): 115–32. https://doi.org/10.1017/S1742058X11000130.

31. Smedley, Brian, Michael Jeffries, Larry Adelman and Jean Cheng. "Race, Racial Inequality and Health Inequities: Separating Myth from Fact." Unnatural Causes. Accessed May 26, 2019. https://www.unnaturalcauses.org/assets/uploads/file/Race_Racial_Inequality_Health.pdf.

32. Lewis, Tené T., Susan A. Everson-Rose, Lynda H. Powell, Karen A. Matthews, Charlotte Brown, Kelly Karavolos, Kim Sutton-Tyrrell, Elizabeth Jacobs, and Deidre Wesley. "Chronic Exposure to Everyday Discrimination and Coronary Artery Calcification in African-American Women: The SWAN Heart Study." *Psychosomatic Medicine* 68, no. 3 (May 2006): 362–68. https://doi.org/10.1097/01.psy.0000221360.94700.16.

33. Lewis, Tené T., Lisa L. Barnes, Julia L. Bienias, Daniel T. Lackland, Denis A. Evans, and Carlos F. Mendes de Leon. "Perceived Discrimination and Blood Pressure in Older African American and White Adults." *The Journals of Gerontology: Series A* 64 no. 9 (September 2009): 1002–8. https://doi.org/10.1093/gerona/glp062.

34. Earnshaw, Valerie A., Lisa Rosenthal, Jessica B. Lewis, Emily C. Stasko, Jonathan N. Tobin, Tené T. Lewis, Allecia E. Reid, and Jeannette R. Ickovics. "Maternal Experiences with Everyday Discrimination and Infant Birth Weight: A Test of Mediators and Moderators Among Young, Urban Women of Color." *Annals of Behavioral Medicine* 45, no. 1 (February 2013): 13–23. https://doi.org/10.1007/s12160-012-9404-3.

35. "Racial/Ethnic Differences in Cardiac Care: The Weight of the Evidence." *The Henry J. Kaiser Family Foundation* (blog), September 29, 2002. https://www.kff.org/disparities-policy/fact-sheet/racialethnic-differences-in-cardiac-care-the-weight/.

SEXISM

36. "Global, Regional, and National Levels of Maternal Mortality, 1990–2015: a systematic analysis for the Global Burden of Disease Study 2015." *The Lancet* 388 (October 8, 2016): 1775-1812. Corrected January 5, 2017. https://www.thelancet.com/pdfs/journals/lancet/PIIS0140-6736(16)31470-2.pdf; "Pregnancy Mortality Surveillance System." Centers for Disease Control and Prevention, August 7, 2018. Accessed January 16, 2019. https://www.cdc.gov/reproductivehealth/maternalinfanthealth/pregnancy-mortality-surveillance-system.htm.

37. "Health Status: Maternal and Infant Mortality." Organization for Economic Co-operation and Development. Accessed February 28, 2019. https://stats.oecd.org/index.aspx?queryid=30116. Updated regularly.

38. Ibid. (Over 63 percent of maternal and infant mortality deaths found to be preventable.)

39. "Pregnancy Mortality Surveillance System." Centers for Disease Control and Prevention.

40. Haskell, Rob. "Serena Williams on Motherhood, Marriage, and Making Her Comeback." *Vogue*, January 10, 2018. https://www.vogue.com/article/serena-williams-vogue-cover-interview-february-2018.

41. Goodwin, Michele "Fetal Protection Laws: Moral Panic and the New Constitutional Battlefront." *California Law Review* 102, no. 4 (August 1, 2014): 781-875. http://scholarship.law.berkeley.edu/california lawreview/vol102/iss4/4.

42. Ibid. at 848.

43. Raymond, Elizabeth G., and David A. Grimes. "The Comparative Safety of Legal Induced Abortion and Childbirth in the United States." *Obstetrics and Gynecology* 119, no. 2 (February 2012): 215–19. https://doi.org/10.1097/AOG.0b013e31823fe923.

44. Gerdts, Caitlin, Loren Dobkin, Diana Greene Foster, and Eleanor Bimla Schwarz. "Side Effects, Physical Health Consequences, and Mortality Associated with Abortion and Birth after an Unwanted Pregnancy." *Women's Health Issues* 26, no. 1 (February 2016): 55–59. https://doi.org/10.1016/j.whi.2015.10.001. https://www.ncbi.nlm.nih.gov/pubmed/26576470.

45. National Women's Health Resource Center, *Forging a Women's Health Research Agenda*. NWHRC. 1990.; Margaret F. Jensvold, Kathleen Reed, David B. Jarrett, and Jean A. Hamilton, "Menstrual Cycle-Related Depressive Symptoms Treated with Variable Antidepressant Dosage," *Journal of Women's Health* 1, no. 2 (June 12, 1992):109–115, 1992. https://www.liebertpub.com/doi/abs/10.1089

/jwh.1992.1.109

46. Lemp, George F., Anne M. Hirozawa, Judith B. Cohen, Pamela A. Derish, Kecin C. McKinney, and Sandra R. Hernandez. "Survival for Women and Men with AIDS." *Journal of Infectious Diseases* 166, no. 1 (July 1992). 74–79. https://www.ncbi.nlm.nih.gov/pubmed/1607710.

47. "Medicaid Enrollment by Gender." *The Henry J. Kaiser Family Foundation* (blog). Accessed December 12, 2017. https://www.kff.org/medicaid/state-indicator/medicaid-enrollment-by-gender/.

POVERTY

48. White, Tracie. "Almost Without Hope" *Stanford Medicine Magazine*, Fall 2013. http://sm.stanford.edu/archive/stanmed/2013fall/article9.html?src=longreads.

49. Ibid.

50. "Indian Health Service Programs–A Retention Analysis." Lewin Group, September 27, 2017. https://aspe.hhs.gov/system/files/pdf/258846/IndianHealthServiceProgramsARetentionAnalysis.pdf.

51. Siddons, Andrew. "The Never-Ending Crisis at the Indian Health Service," *Roll Call*, March 5, 2018. https://www.rollcall.com/news/policy/never-ending-crisis-indian-health-service.

52. Grant, Jaime M., Lisa A. Mottet, and Justin Tanis. *Injustice at Every Turn: A Report of the National Transgender Discrimination Survey.* National Center for Transgender Equality, 2011.https://transequality.org/sites/default/files/docs/resources/NTDS_Report.pdf.

53. "Trans Populations and HIV: Time to End the Neglect." The Foundation for AIDS Research, April 2014. https://www.amfar.org/uploadedFiles/_amfarorg/Articles/On_The_Hill/2014/IB%20Trans%20Population%20040114%20final.pdf.

54. Baral, Stefan, Tonia Poteat, Susanne Strömdahl, Andrea L. Wirtz, Thomas E. Guadamuz, and Chris Beyrer. "Worldwide Burden of HIV In Transgender Women: A Systematic Review and Meta-Analysis." *The Lancet Infectious Diseases* 13, no. 3 (December 21, 2012): 214–22. https://www.ncbi.nlm.nih.gov/pubmed/23260128.

55. Clark, Hollie, Aruna Surendera Babu, Ellen Weiss Wiewel, Jenevieve Opoku, and Nicole Crepaz. "Diagnosed HIV Infection in Transgender Adults and Adolescents: Results from the National HIV Surveillance System, 2009–2014." *AIDS and Behavior* 21, no. 9 (September 2017): 2774–83. https://doi.org/10.1007/s10461-016-1656-7.

56. "HIV and STD Criminal Laws." Centers for Disease Control and Prevention, November 30, 2018. http://www.cdc.gov/hiv/policies /law/states/exposure.html.

57. Hanssens, Catherine, Aish C. Moodie-Mills, Andrea J. Ritchie, Dean Spade, and Urvashi Vaid. "A Roadmap for Change: Federal Policy Recommendations for Addressing the Criminalization of LGBT People and People Living with HIV." New York: Center for Gender & Sexuality Law at Columbia Law School, May 2014. https:// web.law.columbia.edu/sites/default/files/microsites/gender -sexuality/files/roadmap_for_change_full_report.pdf.

58. Arkles, Gabriel. "Safety and Solidarity Across Gender Lines: Rethinking Segregation of Transgender People in Detention", 18 *Temple Political & Civil Rights Law Review* 18, no. 2 (Spring 2009): 515–560. http://archive.srlp.org/files/segregation_Arkles.pdf

59. *In Harm's Way: State Response to Sex Workers, Drug Users, and HIV in New Orleans.* Human Rights Watch, 2013. https://www.hivlawand policy.org/sites/default/files/HRW%20In%20Harm%27s%20 Way%20Report.pdf.

60. "Sex Workers at Risk: Condoms as Evidence of Prostitution in Four US Cities." Human Rights Watch, July 19, 2012. https://www.hrw.org /report/2012/07/19/sex-workers-risk/condoms-evidence-prostitution -four-us-cities.

61. "Hate Violence Against Transgender Communities." National Coalition of Anti-Violence Programs, 2017. https://avp.org/wp-content /uploads/2017/04/ncavp_transhvfactsheet.pdf.

62. Bullard, Robert D., with Paul Mohai, Robin Saha, and Beverly Wright. 2007. "Toxic Wastes and Race at Twenty: 1987–2007." Cleveland: United Church of Christ, 2007. https://www.nrdc.org /sites/default/files/toxic-wastes-and-race-at-twenty-1987-2007.pdf.

63. "Health Status—Infant Mortality Rates." Organisation for Economic Co-operation and Development. Accessed February 28, 2019. http://data.oecd.org/healthstat/infant-mortality-rates.htm.

64. Chandra, Amitabh, Michael Frakes, and Anup Malani. "Challenges To Reducing Discrimination And Health Inequity Through Existing Civil Rights Laws." *Health Affairs* 36, no. 6 (June 2017): 1041–47. https://doi.org/10.1377/hlthaff.2016.1091.

65. Ibid.

66. Rudavsky, Shari. "An Indiana Town Recovering from 190 HIV Cases." *Indianapolis Star*, April 8, 2016. https://www.indystar.com/story/news/2016/04/08/year-after-hiv-outbreak-austin-still-community-recovery/82133598/.

67. Leece, Pamela, Aaron M. Orkin, and Meldon Kahan. "Tamper-Resistant Drugs Cannot Solve the Opioid Crisis." *Canadian Medical Association Journal* 187, no. 10 (July 14, 2015): 717–18. https://doi.org/10.1503/cmaj.150329.

68. Meier, Barry. "Origins of an Epidemic: Purdue Pharma Knew Its Opioids Were Widely Abused." *The New York Times*, May 29, 2018. https://www.nytimes.com/2018/05/29/health/purdue-opioids-oxycontin.html.

69. Ng, Jonathan, and Sean Philip Cotter. "Ex-Pharma CEO Pleads Guilty to Kickbacks to Doctors for Opioid Prescriptions." *Boston Herald*, January 10, 2019. https://www.bostonherald.com/2019/01/09/ex-pharma-ceo-pleads-guilty-to-kickbacks-to-doctors-for-opioid-prescriptions/.

70. Saltzman, Jonathan. "In Rap Video, Insys Opioid Salesmen Boasted of Their Prowess." *Boston Globe*. February 13, 2019. Accessed March 1, 2019. https://www.bostonglobe.com/business/2019/02/13/rap-video-opioid-salesmen-boasted-their-prowess/YsPTTbiDYDq1ZIpEtobmXL/story.html.

71. Frank, Richard G. "Ending Medicaid Expansion Will Leave People Struggling with Addiction without Care." *The Hill*, June 20, 2017.

https://thehill.com/blogs/pundits-blog/healthcare/338579-ending-medicaid-expansion-will-leave-people-struggling-with.

72. McLean, Katherine. "'There's Nothing Here': Deindustrialization as Risk Environment for Overdose."

73. "2015 U.S. Trans Survey." 2015 U.S. Trans Survey. Accessed February 28, 2019. http://www.ustranssurvey.org/.

74. MacDorman, Marian F., and Elizabeth C. W. Gregory. "Fetal and Perinatal Mortality: United States, 2013." *National Vital Statistics Reports* 64, no 8. (July 23, 2015): 1–23. https://www.cdc.gov/nchs/data/nvsr/nvsr64/nvsr64_08.pdf.

75. Mayo Clinic Staff. "Miscarriage—Symptoms and Causes." Mayo Clinic. Accessed February 28, 2019. https://www.mayoclinic.org/diseases-conditions/pregnancy-loss-miscarriage/symptoms-causes/syc-20354298.

76. Buck, Isaac D. "The Cost of High Prices: Embedding an Ethic of Expense into the Standard of Care." *Boston College Law Review* 58, no. 1 (January 31, 2017): 101–150.

77. Huang, Zhihuan Jennifer, Stella M. Yu, and Rebecca Ledsky. "Health Status and Health Service Access and Use among Children in U.S. Immigrant Families." *American Journal of Public Health* 96, no. 4 (April 2006): 634–40. https://doi.org/10.2105/AJPH.2004.049791.

PART VI: WHAT WE DO

1. Hoffman, Beatrix. "Health Care Reform and Social Movements in the United States." *American Journal of Public Health* 93, no. 1 (January 2003): 75–85. https://www.ncbi.nlm.nih.gov/pmc/articles/PMC1447696/

2. Ibid.

3. Reclaim Idaho. "We won the majority of votes in 35 of 44 counties. North, south, east—it didn't matter. Progressive or conservative, rich or poor—it didn't matter. Voters demanded Medicaid Expansion

in every corner of the state. Now it's the job of our legislators to implement full Medicaid Expansion for all 62,000 Idahoans in the coverage gap." Facebook, November 8, 2016. https://www.facebook.com/reclaimidaho/photos/a.680216182180155/958387834362987/?type=3.

4. "Idaho Submits Medicaid Expansion Plan for Federal Review." Associated Press, February 16, 2019. https://www.apnews.com/07c700eb1d8b4337922a28e94c666894

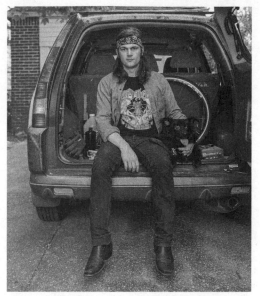

Author photograph by Laura Wing-Kamoosi

ABOUT THE AUTHOR

Timothy Faust's writing has appeared in *Splinter*, *Jacobin*, and *Vice*, among others. He has worked as a data scientist in the healthcare industry, before which he enrolled people in ACA programs in Florida, Georgia, and Texas, where he saw both the shortcomings of the ACA and the consequences of the Medicaid gap firsthand. Since 2017, he's been driving around the United States in his 2002 Honda CR-V talking to people about health inequity in their neighborhoods. He lives in Brooklyn.